A PRACTICAL GU

The Japanese Art of

Reiki

BRONWEN AND FRANS STIENE

Founders of the International House of Reiki, Sydney, Australia

www.reiki.net.au

info@reiki.net.au

BOOKS

Winchester, UK
New York, USA

Copyright © 2005 O Books
O Books is an imprint of John Hunt Publishing Ltd.,
Deershot Lodge, Park Lane, Ropley, Hants, SO24 0BE, UK
office@johnhunt-publishing.com
www.O-books.net

Distribution in:
UK
Orca Book Services
orders@orcabookservices.co.uk
Tel: 01202 665432 Fax: 01202 666219 Int. code (44)

USA and Canada
NBN
custserv@nbnbooks.com
Tel: 1 800 462 6420 Fax: 1 800 338 4550

Australia
Brumby Books
sales@brumbybooks.com
Tel: 61 3 9761 5535 Fax: 61 3 9761 7095

New Zealand
Peaceful Living
books@peaceful-living.co.nz
Tel: 64 7 57 18105 Fax: 64 7 57 18513

Singapore
STP
davidbuckland@tlp.com.sg
Tel: 65 6276 Fax: 65 6276 7119

South Africa
Alternative Books
altbook@global.co.za
Tel: 27 011 792 7730 Fax: 27 011 972 7787

Text: © 2005 Bronwen and Frans Stiene
Design: Jim Weaver Design, Basingstoke, UK
Cover design: Krave Ltd., London

ISBN 978 1 905047 02 4

A CIP catalogue record for this book is available from
the British Library.

Printed and bound by CPI Group (UK) Ltd, Croydon, CR0 4YY

Table of Contents

Appendices

Preface

Our gratitude goes out across the globe to Reiki practitioners everywhere. Without you the Reiki fire would not have been ignited in so many.

Special thanks must also go to those who have directly assisted us with the completion of *The Japanese Art of Reiki*. It feels like a community effort as we have relied on so many to get it to the point of sale in shops. Thank you all for your heartfelt support.

A major part of *The Japanese Art of Reiki* is the artwork. Enormous thanks go to René Geveke and our model Jason Koh. René took photos with such love and creative ability and Jason's patience with us is reflected in his lovely serene features that made him the perfect Reiki model (and, no, he's not Japanese but Singaporean). Thank you, too, to the Cowra Japanese Gardens in New South Wales, Australia for their hospitality in allowing us to take the majority of the photos for this book in their beautiful grounds. Sue Paterson, a big thank you for adjusting photographs with your fabulous can-do attitude.

Donn Pattenden, thank you for your inspired *manga* illustrations. What a blessing that we met you before you escaped to Japan.

Other photos in *The Japanese Art of Reiki* have been sourced from various avenues and we are grateful to each one for their support: BAB books in Japan for allowing us to reproduce photos from Tomita Kaiji's book; the Ittôen community for Tenko san's photo (Fig. 7-1); Tony Henderson for the photos of En No Gyoja (Fig. 1-2) and the shugenja in the Influence of Shugendô; and, finally, Rev. Kuban Jakkoin who kindly offered the photo of shugenja at a cave (Fig. 1-3). Mari Hall and Andy Quan also graciously supplied photos to accompany those taken from Bronwen and Frans Stiene's own collection.

Minamida Tokiko, thank you for your unwavering support. Your laughter mingled with our own on many occasions and we could not have had kinder and more thoughtful help with writing letters in Japanese and translating Japanese words and ways.

Inamoto Hyakuten, a great friend and wonderful teacher. His support and friendship have meant much to us. His sincere offers of help definitely came in handy. You will find his translation of the Meiji Emperor's *waka* in this book.

Other people we must thank are Judith Rabinovitch for her openness and knowledge about Japan and *teate* (hands-on healing) practitioners during the Meiji period; Nevill Drury for supporting us on our path as writers and practitioners; Li Ying for advice and expert knowledge about Ki matters and her superb teaching abilities.

We received editing help from Yani Silvana, Maurizio Floris and Sally Heane. Thank you all for your encouraging words.

Our lovely publisher, John Hunt, deserves great thanks for his support and trust in us. He listens to our ideas with patience and enthusiasm and we have grown to trust his judgment well. Many thanks to his staff, too, for putting this book together and getting it out there.

We must thank our teacher Chris Marsh who gently guides us on our spiritual paths with our personal practice. Thank you, too, to Chris for his translation of the Reiki precepts.

Through Chris Marsh we have had contact with a Japanese nun called Suzuki san (a student of Usui Mikao) and her aide. We thank them both for helping us with our personal practice and answering any technical questions that have supported the historical and philosophical groundwork of *The Japanese Art of Reiki*.

To our students everywhere, thank you for letting us travel with you on your journeys – it is a privilege. You continue to show us the true value of these teachings.

Thank you to our mothers, Elaine and Euk, who have always supported us so selflessly and to Bella who shares her life with "the book".

Usui Mikao, the inspiration for this book and our own spiritual journeys – thank you.

Our many thanks go out to those who have supported *The Reiki Sourcebook* encouraging us to continue our personal and professional journey culminating in *The Japanese Art of Reiki*.

And to you who are reading this right now, may this book guide and inspire you.

Let us begin by writing:

> *mangaichi ayamariga arimashitara goyousha kudasai*
>
> Please forgive us if we've made a mistake.

Introduction

At any given moment, people all over the world are reassessing their life. They wonder if it is worthwhile getting up every morning; if there is any point in going to work, in eating dinner, falling asleep and then getting up to start all over again. They are told they can be anything they want to be and yet they're not even sure what that is.

Ask yourself what you want. Move past the initial expensive car, castle, super job extravaganza and keep asking – what do I want? You may eventually answer: I want to feel good. I want to know who I am. I want to feel free and light without any pressures at all. I want to feel safe and warm and touched by life. I want to know love – unlimited and unconditional. I want to see the beauty around me. I want to experience what this world is all about and understand why I am here.

In short: you want to feel connected. Inside you there is a place that, when accessed, knows what these things feel like. It remembers your connection to life. The system of Reiki will help you find that inner heart and learn from it. You have the aptitude, and the system has the tools. There are no secrets or magic to this, all that is needed is you and your intention to remember. Everyone can find what the Japanese call *honu no reikô*; the spiritual light that exists within.

In the West the word 'Reiki' is understood today to mean both the energy used in the system (spiritual energy) as well as representing the system itself. For the reader's clarity, *The Japanese Art of Reiki* uses the word 'Reiki' to represent the energy used by Reiki practitioners and the words 'system of Reiki' to characterize the system. The term 'practitioner' in this book is used to represent everyone who has learnt the system of Reiki no matter what his or her level, branch or depth of experience.

Many people talk about 'Reiki' as something that they are born with or can do without training. It is true that each person is born with the ability to heal oneself and that spiritual energy flows through each one. The *system* of Reiki on the other hand is a product of the influences of its founder. Not everyone can 'do' Reiki as not everyone has learnt the specific elements that it's system is comprised of. There are many wonderful energetic methods around the world but each one is comprised of its own unique elements and this must be respected.

The founder, Usui Mikao, began his teachings as a spiritual practice for himself – eventually passing this information on to individuals for their own practice. Consequently, *The Japanese Art of Reiki*, focuses solely on self-practice. It is true that if you can look at yourself and work toward healing and making yourself whole, then you naturally affect the world around you. If you really want to help others, taking the healing journey to find out who you are is the first point of call.

The Japanese Art of Reiki offers students a basic historical guideline and, via practical techniques, brings the fundamental Western teachings of hands-on-healing in line with their Japanese origins. This includes pinpointing five basic elements of the system: reducing the system to its fundamental understandings. It is an attempt to bring the Japanese connection back to the system of Reiki, respectfully and truthfully.

This practical book can guide beginners and experienced practitioners alike through the system of Reiki from a Japanese viewpoint. It is suited to every level of practice within the system. The teachings are accessible and written in a manner that allows you to draw on them at different stages of understanding, dependant upon your own level of experience. For this reason *The Japanese Art of Reiki* can be read and re-read many times as your proficiency and knowledge grow.

A beginner will find in this book all the basic information about the system and its practical applications from a traditional Japanese perspective. It is integral though that to learn the system fully, a teacher be employed. *The Japanese Art of Reiki* aims to support you in finding a course, as well as in experimenting with Ki (energy) to gain a greater understanding of where you can go with the system.

Reiki practitioners today are searching for a deeper understanding of the system of Reiki. This book aims to guide practitioners to take the system a step further than what is taught as 'Reiki' in the West. Some teachers in the West do realize this need, and attempt to create follow up courses with new directions. This book, however, does not wish to take you on a different route. It prefers to draw you deep inside the practice you feel you already know by returning you to the philosophy of its roots.

The information in this book has been sourced from various arenas. As teachers of *Usui Reiki Ryôhô*, Frans and Bronwen Stiene were taught and have followed the information that Doi Hiroshi teaches, since the beginning of the 21st century. His connection as a *Usui Reiki Ryôhô Gakkai* member (a traditional Reiki society) has meant that he has had a unique understanding of the system from a Japanese perspective. Frans and Bronwen's interest in Japanese forms continued and they went on to train in Inamoto Hyakuten's *Komyo Reiki Kai*. Inamoto studied with Yamaguchi Chiyoko, a student of Hayashi Chûjirô (student of Usui), before she died in 2003. Other research undertaken by them includes contacting people around the globe who may have known Usui, his students or their students and so on. They have also personally interviewed many Japanese practitioners including a Gakkai member, Yamaguchi, and her son on a visit to Japan. Books from Japanese students of Usui have been examined, such as those from Eguchi and Tomita, along with other relevant Japanese literature. The result of much of this research is also recorded in Bronwen and Frans's research book *The Reiki Sourcebook*. *The Japanese Art of Reiki* uses this information to ground the practitioner in the system so that one's personal Reiki practice is strengthened by knowledge, depth of understanding and clarity of intent.

The authors' personal practice as students of Chris Marsh has given them another understanding of what Usui himself practiced. Chris's teacher is Suzuki san, an old Tendai nun, who studied with Usui. She does not teach Reiki, but an earlier version of Usui's teachings. Suzuki san's personal aide and translator is also a student of these teachings. As this book is about the system of Reiki, Suzuki san's energetic teachings are not in it. Her historical information, though, has been utilized to set the history of the system of Reiki in its place. Some of her philosophical understandings of these earlier teachings that are aligned to those of other traditional Japanese teachers (such as Yamaguchi, Doi and Inamoto) have also been accessed. The backbone of the system is of vital importance to anyone who wishes to study it. It is here that *The Japanese Art of Reiki* takes you beyond a simple book on the subject of 'Reiki'.

The Japanese Art of Reiki is divided into three Parts. Preceding the first Part is a list of the Practices and Techniques incorporated into *The Japanese Art of Reiki*, for easy referral.

Part I takes you on a historical journey of the influences on Usui Mikao. Feel the history and facts rather than learn to recite them – then you will be drawn into the world of Usui. Within this Part you will discover the Japanese energetic system that brings together the energy of the Earth and Heaven to create balance in humankind. Techniques to develop your connection to this energetic system are included. To find out the processes behind learning a Japanese form of Reiki, the imaginary experience of Sato is told. This is a story of a personal crossing over from depression and irregular health to a fresh and more balanced perspective on life. Lastly, thoughts on what healing means according to the basic understanding of the system of Reiki are laid bare.

Part II focuses solely on the five elements of the system of Reiki. These elements are essential traditional self-practice methodology. Without these elements the system that is being taught and practiced is not Reiki. These five elements are: *gokai* (daily precepts), *kokyû hô* (breathing techniques), *tenohira* (palm-healing), *shirushi* and *jumon* (symbols and mantras), and the receiving of *reiju* from a teacher (a blessing from which the Western attunement evolved).

From these elements a multitude of techniques, mantras and symbols have evolved. *The Japanese Art of Reiki* focuses on these traditional practices rather than their modern adaptations. These five basic elements of the system are dissected by looking at what they are, where they came from, how they can benefit you and how you can apply them. Self-probing questions have been included to guide you further into a personal relationship with each element.

In Part III, guidance is offered to help you with the practical rudiments of finding a course to suit your needs and a teacher who can provide support for you on your spiritual path. Also discussed is the setting up of a routine: this will make or break the continuity of your practice. Included are a variety of hints on how to get the most out of your practice and your life.

For ideas on what you can read to supplement your own research and knowledge please refer to the Further Reading section at the back of *The Japanese Art of Reiki*.

There is an art to Reiki and a Japanese one at that. The art grows from a practitioner's hard work and dedication. As with all arts, over time one becomes more skilled as ability develops. The Japanese aspect is integral for a practitioner to make a truthful connection to the origins of this system.

Most people want to know the difference between Western and Japanese Reiki. Obviously the Western form has stemmed from the Japanese and this signifies that some basics will be the same or similar. The name 'Japanese Reiki', as used in *The Japanese Art of Reiki*, does not include the Western or Eastern forms of Reiki that have returned to Japan since the 1980s. Rather, it comprises forms stemming directly from Usui that have not (yet) been influenced by the West. This is a very fine line with the definition constantly being challenged by the effect that Western forms of the system have on many of these traditional forms.

Due to a lack of global standards, however, and a perceived growth in competition by practitioners – Western courses are getting shorter, the number of levels is growing with new marketing techniques, and the 'magic' is getting more unbelievable. The initial Japanese concept of the system is different from what is generally taught in the West today. Not just culturally, but notionally, the most basic understanding of what Reiki is – differs. In the West, the 'Master' or teacher may offer a quick fix: created to get people in and out the door as quickly as possible with a little 'oooh' and 'aaah' along the way. Cures are being promised, diagnosis is instant and wizardry abounds; yet, this is not what the system is about. It is about self-practice, self-responsibility and personal development. Consequently the system of Reiki appears to be losing its integrity through quick and 'easy' courses. Though this concept is enormously appealing to the general public the effect is short lived, ultimately leaving a disappointed and slightly cheated feeling in the student.

The Japanese Art of Reiki will guide you on a journey into the Japanese aspects of this system. It will provide you with historical research and practical techniques to develop your understanding and personal practice. Should you have more questions about this information then do not hesitate to contact the authors through their website www.reiki.net.au.

How to read this book:

- Japanese words are italicized and their translations can be found in the Glossary.
- Japanese names are written with the surname first as is culturally correct.
- The use of upper case is a Western notion and not a Japanese one. When printing Japanese words the authors have taken the liberty of using capitals for people's names and places (in the Western custom) for the reader's added clarity.
- Read this book a couple of times. Let the philosophy seep into you and your approach will naturally become more aligned to the Japanese perspective.

The contents of this book are for general information only. If you wish to learn the system of Reiki it is recommended that you find a teacher that can guide you through the teachings and techniques. The authors do not accept any liability for the use or misuse of any practice or technique in this book.

Japanese Pronunciation:
a is similar to the *a* in father
i is similar to the *ea* in eat
u is similar to the *oo* in look
e is similar to the *e* in egg
o is similar to the *o* in go

(From *An Introduction to Modern Japanese* by Osamu and Nobuko Mizutani.)

List of Practices and Techniques

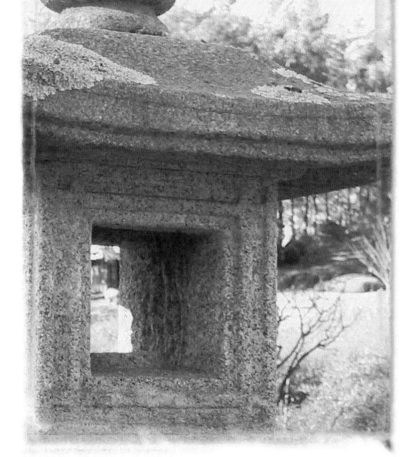

Part I
The Power of Self-healing

1 The Emergence of the System of Reiki

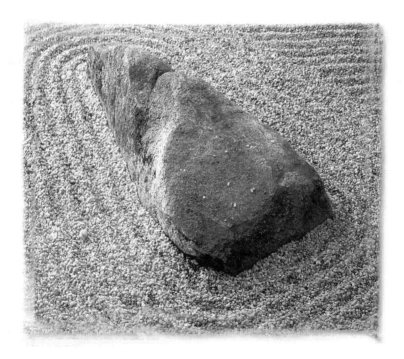

Practitioners of the system of Reiki need to have a solid understanding of the system and the confidence to work within it. An awareness of the roots of the system and how one's practice fits into it will guarantee a practitioner confidence and exceptional skill. This chapter reveals the history of what is known today as the system of Reiki.

Kimonos, Cars and Reiki

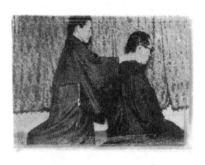

Japan may be famous for its unique craftsmanship, quality automobiles and technological wizardry but it is also fast becoming renowned as the birthplace of the system of Reiki. Over the last century the name Reiki has grown as the system has spread around the globe. The pleasure that millions across the planet have derived from Reiki is in itself inspiring.

Literally translated from the Japanese, Reiki means 'spiritual energy'; it can be described as the energy of everything. To work with this energy is to experience life at its fullest, to be one with all that can be seen and not seen. The system was created to give us this full life experience so that we may remember our connection to life and live in alignment with it. Its creator was a man born into the latter half of the 19th century in Japan, Usui Mikao (Fig. 1–1).

From Japan to the United States of America, around the world and finally back to Japan, this system was developed and buffeted by a multitude of influences. Stemming from a method originally created in the early 1900s to develop an individual's spiritual connection, it returned to Japan at the end of the same century with more worldly

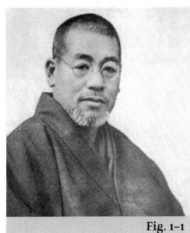

features. Today the system of Reiki is often considered to be many things that its founder would never have dreamed of. The connection to its Japanese roots has been virtually discarded. Now, in the 21st century, and almost a hundred years later, there is a rumbling undercurrent in the global Reiki community: people want to know what the original ideas behind this system were and for whom these teachings

Fig. 1–1   were meant.

The elastic band of connection has been stretched tight, but before it snaps we must bounce back – right back, to the very beginning...

The Beginning

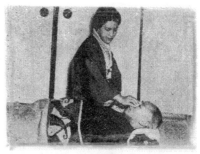

Great social, cultural, economic and technological change occurred in Japan during Usui's lifetime. His birth in 1865 heralded the Meiji Restoration: the opening up of Japan after more than two hundred years of isolation. During this closed historical period there had been a cultural and social intensity in Japan. Foreigners and their accompanying Christianity had been banned. Feudal lords dominated both land and people in a culture that mingled native Shintoism with Buddhism and Taoism (both imported from China and Korea in the 6th century). In Japan's feudal society exquisite handicrafts and perfect manners were valued highly, and religion and martial arts mingled in the same circles.

With the opening up of Japan in the mid-1860s came a national spiritual transformation. Industrialization, urbanization and improvements in public transport are named by researcher Inoue Mobutaka[1] as the cause for change in the social foundation of Japan. From the traditional ways of maintaining faith systems in a closed society with very little mobility, this opening up threatened the family and village unit. Parents could no longer be assured that their children would continue to follow in their footsteps, not just vocationally but also spiritually. New religions and spiritual groups began to emerge all over Japan to compensate for this sense of disconnection in people's lives. People 'afflicted with the feeling of alienation and deprivation in an industrialized society' felt that these new spiritual methods offered them a form of salvation.[2]

This national search for inner connectedness and meaningful spirituality was likely to have also been an inspiration for Usui Mikao. He drew from his own spiritual experiences to evolve a teaching that he believed would benefit everyone – whether they were religious or not.

Self-healing

Usui's method appears not to have been to teach new things, but rather to help practitioners to break down their accumulated old patterns and 'bad habits'. In this way practitioners would gradually discover their true nature and realise that inherently each human is the keeper of all the knowledge that he or she requires.

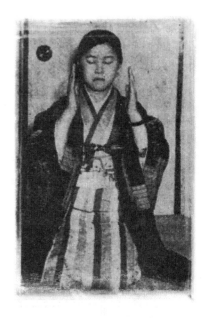

The basic premise of this method is that healing exists *within* each person, not outside, and therefore the essence of the teachings is self-practice. The ultimate healing tool is the practitioner's own dedication to healing the self: another can never give this depth of healing.

Suzuki san, born in 1895 and still alive at the time of writing, claims that the teachings assume people are already spiritual in nature and are used to help practitioners become 'entirely human'. The first teaching of Usui that was given to students, she states, was the five precepts or *gokai*. Later came meditations and/or mantras for students to practice in an ongoing teacher/student based relationship. Suzuki san said that Usui became renowned as a healer later in life and that his initial teachings (his own practice) were based on the concept of reconnecting to one's spirituality. Students found that they experienced healing from his teachings and his practices. Usui performed a 'spiritual blessing' or *reiju* on his students. This was the forerunner to what is known as an attunement today. The *reiju* is not to attune/empower or transform someone, but is merely a blessing of a spiritual nature.[3] What was taught at this time appears to have been based strongly on traditional Japanese cultural and religious mores.

Influence of Tendai Mikkyô

A major influence on Usui was religion. This does not mean that the system of Reiki is a religion – it is not. Usui was extremely smart in that he brought together elements from the many influences in his life to create something that could be practiced by anyone without the trappings of religion. Unlike in the West, where one religion is considered more than enough, the Japanese draw on many

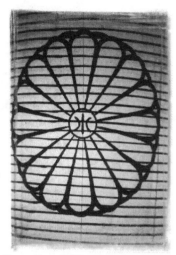

religions to cover their needs. To confirm the difference between religion and a spiritual practice: a religion typically has a priesthood, central deity and a dogmatic belief system. A spiritual practice has none of these and is guided by personal experience.[4]

Chris Marsh, a student of Suzuki san, states that Usui's original teachings were mostly Mikkyô made accessible to the everyday person as Usui's teachings cover the same ground that Mikkyô does. Mikkyô is known as 'esoteric Buddhism' and is an esoteric[5] arm of Tendai Buddhism. Tendai is based on the belief that the Lotus Sutra[6] is Buddha's complete and perfect teaching: it includes meditations based on esoteric foundations. These foundations were originally brought across from China and were honed to adjust to Japanese concepts. Today some branches of the system of Reiki try to incorporate Chinese Buddhist thoughts or, strangely, Tibetan Buddhist thoughts, into the practice. Though Japanese Buddhism may have come from China initially, it is a different system, having been affected by almost 1500 years of Japanese culture and native belief systems such as Shintoism. Tibetan Buddhism did not directly influence Japanese Buddhism as both countries were introduced to it from China at the same time. This is not to say that some correlations do not exist between Buddhism from countries other than Japan – very basic Buddhist interpretation is similar across the globe. Paul Varley, author of *Japanese Culture*, writes that, 'the Japanese, within the context of a history of abundant cultural borrowing from China in pre-modern times and the West in the modern age, have nevertheless retained a hard core of native social, ethical and cultural values by means of which they have almost invariably molded and adapted foreign borrowing to suit their own tastes and purposes.[7]

Only a couple of years ago there were still twelve students of Usui alive, some as old as a hundred and twelve, including monks, one nun and a farmer. At the time of writing *The Japanese Art of Reiki* just five of these students are left, according to Suzuki san, though teachers are being trained to ensure continuity for these unique teachings.

Living students of Usui state that he was taught in a temple school and continued his Buddhist education to the point where he was known as a lay Tendai priest (*zaike*). Therefore he would have had an understanding of these 'secret' Mikkyô esoteric practices. By the term 'secret' it is understood that students receive what their teacher believes *benefits* their practice rather than *confuses* it.

In his book, *Zen in the Art of Archery*, Eugen Herrigel explains this process. As a beginner his teacher gave him a very stiff bow to work with. He found it almost impossible to open his bow correctly until one day his teacher taught him a breathing technique and suddenly everything became easy. His teacher explained, 'If from the very start I had taught you the breathing exercises, you would have found them unnecessary. Now you will believe what I tell you and practice as if it were really important.'[8]

Teaching one aspect of a practice at a time appears to be a common Japanese method of instruction. In Usui's early teachings, students are asked to practice a certain technique until the teacher can see that they are ready to move on. Different techniques are given to individuals depending on their background and experiences.

Influence of Shintoism

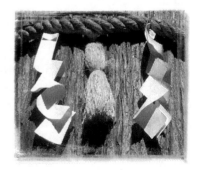

Shinto is the indigenous faith of the Japanese people and is as old as the culture itself. The *kami*, or gods, are the objects of worship in Shinto. *Kami* may be birds, animals, mountains, trees or people. The following definition was given by an 18th century scholar, Motoori Norinaga (1730–1801): 'According to ancient usage, whatever seemed strikingly impressive, possessed the quality of excellence, or inspired a feeling of awe was called *kami*.'[9]

Shinto has no founder and no sacred scriptures; in fact Shintoism did not even have a name until Buddhism was imported in the 6th century (consequently acquiring one to make itself distinguishable). Buddhism has incorporated some Shinto concepts to create a typical Japanese flavor quite separate from Chinese Buddhism.

Buddhism lost governmental support with the advent of the Meiji Restoration in 1873. The new regime attempted to control religion and the population by supporting Shintoism against Buddhism. Consequently Shintoism became the state religion. Once any other form of organized religion became too large (and there were many at this time) they either had to bow to the Shinto template or disband. However, there was no restriction of individual belief and practice as long as no effort was made to influence others. In this, Usui's early teachings remained safe. 'Usui did not see himself as a teacher. He made no claims for what he practiced – others approached him and asked to learn. That is how he was free to do as he did.'[10] What he taught was also not a religion, yet any spiritual teacher with a following may well have run the risk of being restricted.

During this period Suzuki san became a Tendai Buddhist nun. Of the decision for her to become a Buddhist nun she has said that it was an 'extremely difficult' time. Her family practiced a mixture of both Shintoism and Buddhism as was quite common in Japan. Born in 1895 she was just fourteen when her husband to be was killed in battle, leaving her to become a nun. On practicing Buddhism during this mono-religious period she said of her own Buddhist practice that, 'There were only a small number of communities which were allowed to operate openly'. Once Suzuki san reached the age of twenty in 1915, it was acceptable to her current teacher that she study formally with Usui, a distant relative. She has said that '*Sensei*[11] shared what he knew all his adult life. There was no fixed point at which he began to teach. People were drawn to him because of his charisma and wisdom, and asked him to teach them, he never placed himself in the role of teacher.' The approximate time that he began to bring his teachings together was around 1912 to 1914.[12] Notes with some precepts (*gokai*), meditations, and poems (*gyosei*) written by the Emperor of the time, were given to Usui's students around 1920.

A Shinto practitioner called Eguchi Toshihiro also influenced Usui. According to Professor J. Rabinovitch[13], 'Eguchi was a student of Usui sensei's for about two years and a close personal friend for much longer'. The Professor goes on to say that 'since Eguchi in particular studied under Usui with such seriousness, his writings are especially valuable in tracing early proto-Reiki and better understanding the Buddhist and spiritual underpinnings of hand healing.' She states records and a journal of Eguchi's, detailing information about his relationship with Usui, have survived the decades.

It would be easy to say that Usui's teachings evolved solely from Shinto and Mikkyô practices but that is not the case. Some elements also belonged to martial arts and a mysterious practice called Shugendô.

Influence of Martial Arts

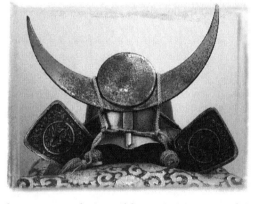

As the cities swelled during the Meiji Restoration various groups of people, including unemployed *samurai*, came together. The *samurai* were obsolete under the Meiji regime and were ordered to cut off their topknots and to remove their emblematic 'two swords'. These topknots and swords were symbolic codes of dress that displayed the high status of *samurai* in Japanese society.

Samurai had held positions of power under the *shôgun* (prior to the Meiji Restoration) as protectors and guardsmen, while commoners, the majority of the population, had lived without the right to vote or own a surname. Usui's family was *hatamoto samurai*[14], a privileged rank who had worked as the personal guard of the *shôgun*. Samurai, were taught and practiced martial arts from a very young age.

Depending upon an individual's region and clan of origin, the skills that each *samurai* clan practiced were unique.

Martial artists, often thought of as ruffians at the beginning of the 1900s, grew in stature as a formalization of styles emerged. Previously unemployed martial artists moved to the cities and began teaching and creating modern forms of martial arts. Some of these styles, like *judo* and *karate*, were very physical, while others, such as *aikidô*, were more spiritual and contemplative in nature. Usui's *samurai* ancestors were the once influential Chiba clan and as an expert martial artist himself, Usui trained in *aiki jutsu*, which was popularized by Takeda Sokaku. Takeda is renowned as the teacher of the founder of *aikidô*, Ueshiba Morihei. *Aiki jutsu* includes many physical skills but it also 'involves harmonizing with Ki' and 'can transform the lives of its participants' according to H.E. Davey, author of *Living the Japanese Arts and Ways*. Through this form 'it is possible to experience enhanced calmness, concentration, willpower and physical fitness in daily living'.[15] The early teachings of Usui included elements of his martial arts training, later developing into the system of Reiki.[16] Suzuki san has said about the influence of martial arts on Usui's teachings that, 'It would be true to say that his training showed him glimpses of other ways and perhaps opened doors for him to study further.'

In tracing back the elements of Usui's teachings, similar elements are found in more than one area that influenced him (such as Mikkyô and martial arts). Researchers today say that though there is a similarity of names utilized in both martial arts and Japanese religious practices (such as the word 'esoteric') the intent or aim is often altered. A practice takes on its own unique purpose according to the environment it is practiced in. Buddhist and Shinto ethics have naturally influenced Japanese culture (as has Christianity influenced Western cultures) so it is only natural that their influence be found in Japanese martial arts. It has been suggested that Mikkyô type practices found their way into the hands of the martial artists via the traveling monks and mountain monks. These monks would teach specific mudras (symbolic hand or body positions) and meditations or visualizations to those in need (such as the Ninja clans).This influence was reciprocated between the two groups resulting in the seemingly incongruent existence of meditating Ninjas and so-called 'warrior monks' (popularly called *yamabushi* today).

Influence of Shugendô

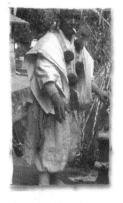

En no Ozunu (En no Gyôja) (Fig. 1–2) is the legendary founder of Shugendô. He practiced esoteric Buddhism on Mt Katsuragi from the year 666 for more than thirty years until he attained miraculous powers. This experience led to the creation of esoteric mountain Buddhism that became formalized during the late 8th century and early 9th century in Japan.

According to Miyake Hitoshi's book, *Shugendô*, the mixture of ancient religious beliefs and practices in the mountains were influenced by shamanism[17], Shintoism, Taoism and Buddhism. Practitioners of Shugendô became known as *yamabushi* or *shugenja*. He also writes that, 'some people entered the holy spiritual regions of the mountains and performed ascetic practices under the guidance of 'mountain men'. These people were able to draw on the power of the *kami* and became religious figures who performed magico-religious activities. The ascetics of the esoteric Buddhist Shingon and Tendai traditions are representative of these figures. During the Heian period (794–1185), people who had cultivated such practices and attained magical powers were called *shugenja*. This marks the beginning of Shugendô as a distinct religious tradition.'[18]

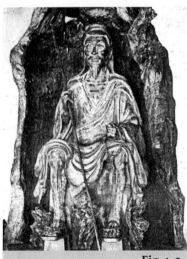

There are many famous mountains in Japan related to Shugendô. Its most influential form was found in 'the three mountains of Kumano' and this branch became known as the Honzanha. A large number of *shugenja* gathered in the Kumano area and were active there throughout history. Their practice on the mountains involved using magico-powers, according to Miyake, to heal disease. Other roles undertaken by

Fig. 1–2

them were 'offering religious services such as fortune-telling and divination (*bokusen*), obtaining oracles through mediums, prayers or ritual incantation (*kitô*) and exorcism (*chôbuku*).'[19] *Shugenja* were required by family clans to heal disease and to aid in the avoidance of misfortune.

Usui is believed to have practiced as a *shugenja* as well as a Tendai Buddhist, completing mountain practices on at least two Japanese mountains (Fig. 1–3). Suzuki san names Mt Hiei (*hiei zan*), a famous Tendai mountain, as one where old sutra copies exist with Usui's Buddhist name of Gyoho or Gyo-tse on them. Mt Kurama (*kurama yama*) is the other, with its link to Usui related on Usui's memorial stone[20] at a Pure Land Buddhist temple[21] in Tôkyô. The memorial stone states that in 1922 Usui received divine inspiration while fasting on Mt Kurama. Fasting is common practice amongst ascetics and *shugenja* along with the use of cold water (think mountains and waterfalls in the middle of a freezing Japanese winter) and the recitation of words of power. Carmen Blacker, author of the renowned book *The Catalpa Bow*, writes that these three *gyô* (ascetic

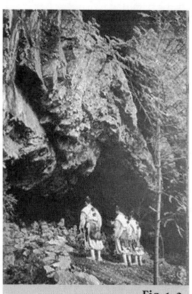

Fig. 1–3

practices) are the means to build up 'a store of power which can then be channeled into the required direction.'[22]

The Meiji regime outlawed Shugendô in 1872 because of Shugendô's mix of Buddhism and Shintoism. The government required that branches of Shugendô belonged to the Buddhist religions of either Tendai or Shingon. Shugendô's Honzanha sect elected to join Tendai. After this disbandment many *shugenja* continued with their practices under the guise of traditional religion. This may well have been the case for Usui who, though he practiced as a *shugenja*, was also known as a lay Tendai priest. Due to the outlawing of Shugendô many new religions sprang up 'to take its place and respond to the human need for fulfilling worldly aspirations'.[23] Shugendô thus became the central foundation for many of these new religions. After World War II, the Religious Corporation Ordinance was enacted in Japan and many religious organizations, such as Shugendô, became independent once again.

Suzuki san and other monks and nuns were attracted to Usui's teachings because they could see what he had done – he had brought together 'the Mystery of the Hidden Teachings of Tendai (Mikkyô) and the teachings of the Shugendô monks'. To understand why this is exceptional is to know that it takes between fifteen and twenty years to complete the Mikkyô teachings and a further fifteen to twenty years to get anywhere near the Shugendô teachings. He brought the core of both together and presented them as a possibility for someone to attain within a lifetime.[24]

After Usui's experience on Mt Kurama in 1922 he set up an official seat of learning in Tôkyô. These latter teachings were not apparently solely focused on an individual's spiritual purification but also on a previously limited aspect of Usui's teachings – palm-healing.

Influence of New Sects[25], Movements and Groups

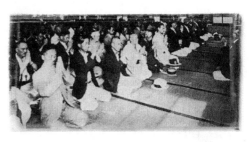

Usui was not the only person to be interested in spiritual matters and developing methods for both religious practitioners and laymen to experience enlightenment. There was a significant movement during the late 1800s and early 1900s that included the practice of palm-healing. This was either called by the generic term, *teate*, or when referring to a structured form of palm-healing as *tenohira*. Palm-healing has always been a part of religious life. Monasteries often include a room called an *enjudo*, a life-preserving hall, where healing, including forms of palm-healing, takes place.

Usui was a member of the now almost mythical *Rei Jutsu Kai*, an association known as the spiritual powerhouse of modern Japan. Its aim was to maintain the essence of the old ways (pre-Meiji restoration) without necessarily holding on to one specific tradition. These spiritual teachers, all originating from varied backgrounds such as Tendai, Shingon, Zen, Jodo shu, Shinto and even Christianity, would meet a number of times a year.[26]

At first when the West forced its way into Japan in the 1860s, Western culture was embraced. The West held an allure for the Japanese, culturally as well as spiritually. In the West, at this time, spiritual practices with new philosophies, such as the Theosophical Society co-founded by Helen Blavatsky, were popular. These spiritual philosophies sparked curiosity in the Japanese, but by the 1880s there was to be a complete turn around. Conservative viewpoints abounded with many Japanese wishing to return to and retain their traditional ways.[27] This traditionalist period transpired in Usui's early adult life and may have influenced him and his interest in traditional Japanese ways. It has been thought that Usui's practices may also have been an attempt to try to keep these ancient practices (such as the banned Shugendô) alive under a hostile regime.

Chris Marsh relates that Usui was well known for his spiritual practice but less well known as a palm-healer. There were a great many other groups during this period that focused solely on *teate*. A few of the more famous groups that grew during these periods and who practiced *teate* within a spiritual framework are the *Ittôen* community, Tenrikyô, Oomoto and Sekai Meshiakyô. Mochizuki Toshitaka lists numerous spiritual groups that evolved during the early 20th century in his Japanese book, *Iyashi No Te*[28].

It is curious that for a country like Japan experiencing such spiritual revolutions there was also a strong militaristic pull. The common people had stepped out of a serf-like culture into one of relative freedom (one at least including voting rights) only to become nationalistic slaves within the navy and army. Nearer to the end of his life Usui was invited by naval officers to teach them palm-healing to use as 'first aid' on naval vessels. This particular branch of the teachings still exists today in the form of the Japanese *Usui Reiki Ryôhô Gakkai*.

Carmen Blacker names the beginning of the Meiji Restoration, 1860s, and the 1920s and 30s as two major periods where there was a boom in new sects, movements and groups in Japan with culturally shamanistic qualities.[29]

Hayashi Chûjirô, a retired naval officer and surgeon, studied with Usui in 1925. It is believed that it was his technical knowledge that helped create a student manual that listed body parts and illnesses with corresponding hand positions. Around this time symbols were also added to the teachings to aid the inexperienced naval personnel in sensing energy.

In 1926, Usui Mikao died of a stroke leaving behind his wife, Suzuki Sadako, and a boy, Fuji (born in 1908), and a girl, Toshiko (born in 1913).

Beyond Usui Mikao

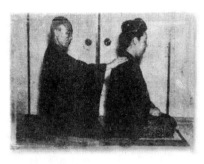

The four major influences on Usui of Tendai Mikkyô, Shintoism, martial arts and Shugendô formed Usui's personal practice (Fig. 1–4). From this he adjusted and altered the teachings until finally formalizing them: making them accessible to even those inexperienced with energy work.

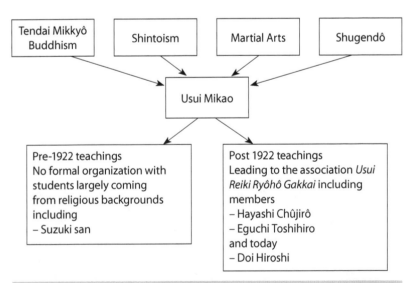

Fig. 1–4   Influences on Usui Mikao and his resulting teachings

Usui's earlier spiritual students, Chris Marsh relates, went back to their monasteries and homes after Usui's death. They continued with their practice without the apparent need of an official teaching infrastructure.

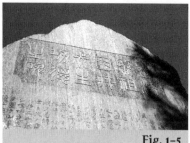

Fig. 1–5

On the other hand he states that the society called the *Usui Reiki Ryôhô Gakkai* was created as a memorial to Usui after his death with Usui's name being recorded as the first president of the association in a gesture of commemoration (Fig. 1–5). The *Usui Reiki Ryôhô Gakkai* was set up in various cities throughout Japan.[30] Members would come together on a regular basis (often weekly) to practice techniques under the guidance of the head teachers or *shihan*.

Eguchi Toshihiro (Fig. 1–6) initially joined the *Usui Reiki Ryôhô Gakkai* in 1927. He left within two years because he found their fees too high (high fees are quite common in Japanese associations) and he did not entirely agree with elements of the teachings.[31] He went on to set up the *Tenohira Ryôji Kenkyû Kai* (Palm-healing Research Centre) and became a famous palm-healer. He wrote many books and taught scores of students.

Another student of Usui, Tomita Kaiji (Fig. 1–7), taught over 200,000 students palm-healing, also writing books on the subject.

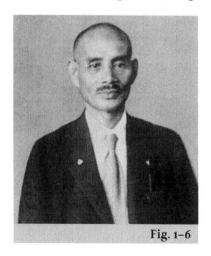

Fig. 1–6

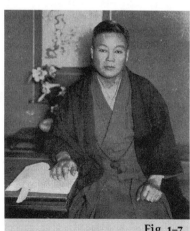

Fig. 1–7

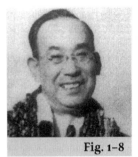
Fig. 1–8

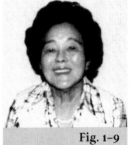
Fig. 1–9

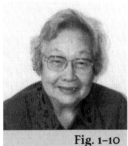
Fig. 1–10

Hayashi (Fig. 1–8) practiced under the auspices of the *Usui Reiki Ryôhô Gakkai* until the early 1930s when he officially opened his own centre called the *Hayashi Reiki Kenkyû Kai* (Hayashi's Spiritual Energy Research Society). Hayashi appears to have developed the first actual commercial center where paying clients could come to receive healing and practitioners would work on them. Hayashi wrote that he had taught thirteen Reiki teachers by 1938.

From 1936–1938 Hawayo Takata (Fig. 1–9), an American-born Japanese woman, studied with him and became one of these Reiki teachers. Another known student of Hayashi was Yamaguchi Chiyoko[32] (Fig. 1–10) who, until her passing in 2003, taught in Kyôto with her son Tadao. Other members of Yamaguchi's family were also teachers and practitioners along with Hayashi's wife, Chie[33], and a man called Tatsumi[34]. These more practical palm-healing teachings that Takata was taught are what developed in the West and have come to be known as the system of Reiki today.

Influence of the West

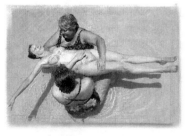

Takata took the system of Reiki to Hawaii (USA) in 1938 and set up the first foreign Reiki clinic and school. It seems that what she taught technically was in line with Hayashi's teachings. Like Hayashi, she did not teach the chakra system. Instead, her diary relates that she knew of and was taught about the *hara* method. Her historical recollections of the system of Reiki on the other hand varied according to when they were told.

Hayashi Chûjirô committed suicide in 1940 by cutting an artery.[35] His wife continued teaching in his place.

By the mid-1970s Hawayo Takata realized that she needed students to whom she could pass on her teachings. She trained twenty-two teacher students to teach the system of Reiki as she knew it. During Takata's time there were still people quietly practicing in Japan who had been taught by Usui and his students. These practitioners appear to have had no inclination to contact the strands of the system that were being practiced in the West at that time.

Hawayo Takata died of a heart attack in 1980. After she died her students began to set up their own practices and create Reiki groups and associations. Perhaps due to a lack of infrastructure, or the sudden rise of the New Age movement, or because Takata's formidable influence was no longer present, debate began over what was the true system of Reiki. A group called the Reiki Alliance standardized the Western system and taught what they called *Usui Shiki Ryôhô*. Hawayo Takata's granddaughter, Phyllis Lee Furumoto, was their head and the term 'Grandmaster' was introduced to reflect her position. This term had not been used previously in the system of Reiki in either Japan or the West.

Barbara Weber Ray, another Reiki teacher student of Hawayo Takata, began her own system, calling it *The Radiance Technique*. She gradually created seven levels instead of three and claimed to have the only true teachings. These teachings appear to have been influenced by her New Age beliefs.

Other students, including Iris Ishikuro and her student Arthur Robertson, incorporated more New Age concepts into the system of Reiki during the 1980s. It was at this point that mythological Tibetan teachings entered the scene. People began to channel information from spirits and guides in a New Age format and the system of Reiki took on a new life, quite different from its Japanese origins.

The Full Circle

This Westernized system called Reiki returned to Japan in the 1980s and its modern hands-on-healing based teachings have become very popular with the Japanese, just as they have in the West. It was not until the mid-1990s that Western researchers began to unearth indications that traditional practitioners of Usui's teachings were still alive.

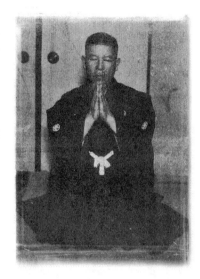

The new millennium has brought with it a gradual opening up by the Japanese community. Some of the older non-Westernized teachings of Usui that have come to the light include:

- *Usui Reiki Ryôhô Gakkai* – one member, Doi Hiroshi, has received permission to reveal some information about the society. He has been teaching Westerners since 1999 in branches such as *Usui Reiki Ryôhô* and his own Western hybridization, *Gendai Reiki Hô*. Although World War II had almost brought the society to a halt it gradually picked up again. Today it is still a practicing society, although on a much smaller scale than when it began in the 1920s and 30s.
- Yamaguchi Chiyoko, a student of Hayashi Chûjirô, died in 2003 but left her teachings with her son, Tadao, and Inamoto Hyakuten. Other family members had studied with Hayashi and it was not until her later years that she began to teach and pass these teachings on.
- Suzuki san is one of five students of Usui still alive at the time of writing (aged a hundred and nine) that is trained to a teacher level. A distant cousin of Usui's wife and a nun since the age of fourteen, she trained formally with Usui for five years. She is still teaching today and considers the only similarities between the system of Reiki (as it is known today) and Usui's early teachings to be Usui himself.

This rekindling of interest in these older teachings has meant that Reiki students have begun tracing their lineages[36] and what they have been taught back to Usui. Some have found that what they know of as the system of Reiki no longer bears much semblance to Usui's or even Hayashi's or Takata's teachings. Symbols, mantras, histories, attunements and even fundamental beliefs about spiritual energy may vary. A very few systems have even been concocted with false histories to satisfy some perverse human need. For all of these reasons it is especially grounding for practitioners to learn and integrate the system's Japanese heritage into their practice. In this way the future of Reiki and its benefits are assured of reaching people all over the world.

2 The Three Diamonds

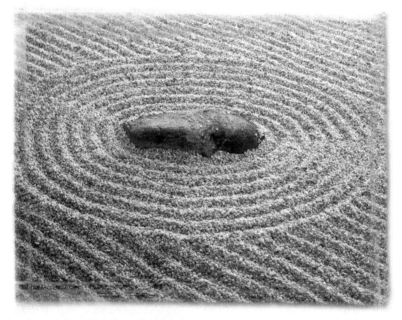

In describing Usui's early teachings, Suzuki san says, 'What people consider to be life is merely existence – survival. Living, *really living*, is what you learn.'

Suzuki san should know. At the age of a hundred and nine, this Tendai nun travels the world, spends time recalling the details of her life with her biographer, teaches, and still practices Usui's teachings. Although she now enjoys having more quiet time in her life she is said to be in an astonishing state of good health for her advanced age.

In Japan to be in a fine state of health translates as being good or vigorous in spirit (*genki*), while a weakened state of health is thought of as a decline or loss in spirit. The underlying notion here is that the wellspring of life is located in one's spirit.

Usui's early teachings work with the spirit. Although the focus of the system of Reiki appears to have developed into one of palm-healing only, the initial premise of spiritual development can center a modern student's practice. A solid understanding of the system is reflected in the practitioner's desire to work on him or herself and the results achieved from this dedicated practice.

To see what can be achieved by working with the system of Reiki it is wise to first find out what Usui thought about the concept of spiritual energy.

Ki

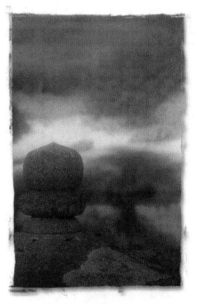

There are hundreds of expressions in the Japanese language that use the word Ki. Ki, when translated philosophically, is often described as 'energy', 'universal energy' or 'life force energy'.

As explained previously it may also be applied to express the condition of one's health, and is even used to convey one's disposition, manner or character. Its origin is Chinese, and the word arrived in Japan with the early Chinese Buddhist texts during the 6th century. In China, Ki is pronounced as *chi* (also written as *qi*) and is commonly found in the names of Chinese energetic arts such as *qi gong* (Ki cultivation).

The word Rei from Reiki can be defined as 'sacred' or 'spiritual'. Thus one reading of Reiki might be 'sacred energy' or 'spiritual energy'. This definition places the energy used in the system of Reiki in context. This energy is not separate to Ki – it is simply the system's name for Ki. Therefore the word Reiki can be considered to be a reverent form of the word Ki.

But what is Ki? This is an energy that cannot be measured or contained, although it can be cultivated and experienced. To understand the concept of cultivating one's Ki imagine a vegetable patch. Regular tending and caring for this garden is a necessity if one wishes to achieve vigorous and plentiful growth. If the weeds and rocks are allowed to strangle new growth or do not allow direct sunlight there will be no progress. In fact in the long run this vegetable patch that held so much promise may become a jungle of confusion or a barren landscape. Each effort, no matter how small, to work on this garden affects the outcome. Humans, too, must tend to themselves by practicing their techniques. No matter how small the effort their lives will be affected, allowing Ki to flow more freely and easily through them. It is at this point that the experience of Ki cultivation occurs.

Tendai belief has it that there is a great pool of Ki from which energy is drawn to create new life and existence. This concept alludes to the inbuilt belief of Oneness or wholeness of everything. We all come from the same One and return to that One. When Suzuki san talks of becoming 'entirely human', this concept may also be described as experiencing Oneness. There are many signs that indicate a growing connection with Oneness in our lives. It is also possible to notice where the challenge of disconnection lies (Fig. 2–1).

Oneness	Disconnectedness
Patience	Impatience
Calm	Anger
Acceptance	Disappointment
Inner Knowledge	Ignorance
Humility	Arrogance

Fig. 2–1 Signs of Oneness

If it is recognized that all creation is formed from this same one source, then there is an immediate sense of connection to life. Each animal, mountain, lake, building, plastic object, car, planet or person shares a common essence. This essence, Ki, is as unlimited as the sky that stretches past the horizon.

Think of this – one cannot connect to energy because the connection is already there. At any time that the word connection is used it is in fact referring to your connection to yourself. Everything, animate and inanimate, pulses with the rhythm of the universe.

The term universe does not indicate solely the universe that is technically lived in (the solar system etc.) but everything that can be understood and not understood. It includes existence and non-existence, all thoughts and things not yet thought about. This is the universe.

Ki Components

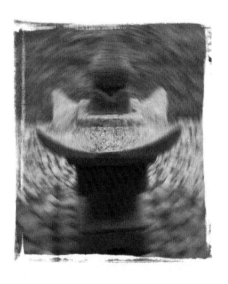

Two primary components of the universe are Earth Ki and Heaven Ki.

As Usui was a Shugendô practitioner it is ideal to become acquainted with its early cosmology. One cosmological theory states that through the union of the dual forces of Earth Ki and Heaven Ki all things were born.[37] Consequently, it is believed that humans are a blend of both these components. Therefore, for a human to achieve a state of equanimity in life, these elements need to become balanced with one another.

Earth Ki is representative of the physical form while Heaven Ki signifies the mind. The integration of mind and body is a typically Japanese concept. To see the connection of these two and how they integrate know that the body reflects the mind. How you feel and think is expressed through your physical posture and actions. By simply *thinking* of the Earth Ki point (about 3 inches or 8cm below the navel) – the mind is integrated with the body. This is due to the mind instantly focussing on a point that exists in the Now – your physical self. Unlike your mind – that which races to and fro from thought to new thought – the physical body is captured in the present. This simple action is therefore extremely beneficial for the mind. It gives it a sense of the Now, drawing it back from its journeys to the past and future into an awareness of this exact moment in time.

Joining together, the mind and body not only create a sense of balance but stimulate a third primary component of Ki – Heart Ki. This triune can be though of as the three diamonds. A diamond is often used as an analogy of the self in Buddhism. Each and every day a practitioner polishes the diamond by performing his or her practice. This is a constant task for humans who, in this earthly realm, attract dirt: becoming muddy and tarnished. A diamond is so sharp that it can cut through almost anything humanity attaches itself to, bringing back the true essence of life as seen in the perfection of a sparkling diamond.

The three diamonds of Earth Ki, Heaven Ki and Heart Ki are at the foundation of the system of Reiki. They are also at the crux of many facets of Japanese culture, religion and philosophy.

Ki, with its energetic components of Earth, Heaven and Heart, is categorically Japanese (originating in China) and relates directly to the Japanese system of Reiki, unlike the Indian Chakra energy system which was adapted to the modern system of Reiki during the popularity of the New Age movement in the 1980s and 1990s.

Once teachers and practitioners in the West connect this understanding of the Japanese use of Ki with their own practice, they will gain a deeper level of comprehension, progress and satisfaction.

Though the three diamonds are described as having a distinct physical home in the body, the energy still radiates throughout the entire being and is not restricted by the physicality of the body. Whether it be the awareness of Earth, Heaven or Heart Ki, these energies may be felt throughout the whole body.

Discussing 'energies' as separate entities here is quite distinct from many Western descriptions of energy. These individual components of Ki are a part of the whole (Ki) but will naturally exist at different levels of intensity unless one is completely balanced.

All individual experience of energy is subjective and no one can tell another what to feel, how to feel it or how much is felt. These experiences are only relative to the practitioner and cannot be compared to those experienced by other individuals.

At this point it is useful for the reader to gain a better understanding of what is meant by the terms Ki, Earth Ki, Heaven Ki and Heart Ki. An energetic awareness of these essential underpinnings to the system of Reiki will aid the reader when working through Part II of *The Japanese Art of Reiki*.

The three diamonds will merely remain concepts until they are experienced. Words cannot explain that which can only be realized through practice. Therefore techniques are included to help readers achieve their own personal understanding of each component. Combining the reading of the text with an actual practice will eventuate in a clearer and fuller understanding of these fundamental concepts. The following techniques are taken from various energetic backgrounds to support the reader's understanding of the three diamonds and are not traditional Usui or 'Reiki' techniques.

Balancing the three diamonds is the general focus of many techniques taught both in Japan and China. As all aspects of the human experience are interlinked, even practicing a simple technique can generate a wealth of inner change for a person. This book, however, does not attempt to be a substitute for working with a qualified teacher.

Sensing Ki Technique

An elementary technique to bring awareness to energy or Ki is to create an energy ball. This simple technique offers budding practitioners of all ages the chance to feel for themselves the movement of energy and its many effects.

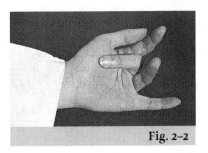

Fig. 2–2

Standing or sitting, rub your hands together. This action creates a movement of blood and energy in the hands and increases sensitivity. To find the point where energy emanates from the hand let your fingers drop into your palm. You will find that the tip of your middle finger naturally falls onto this energetic point (Fig. 2–2). Gently stimulate this point by rubbing it with the thumb of your other hand. Swap hands and repeat.

Create between your hands a make-believe ball about the size of a small basketball (Fig. 2–3). Make sure your hands are relaxed and flexible, easily creating a ball-like shape. Throughout the rest of this technique your hands do not physically touch.

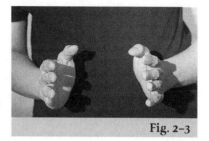

Fig. 2–3

Slowly bring your hands in and out, changing the shape of the ball from the basketball to a tennis ball and back out again to a basketball. As your hands roll the ball around freely, enjoy the sensation of holding this energetic creation.

Now bring your awareness to your hands – is there a tingling, a warmth, a magnetic pull or something unique to you? Experience it for what it is – an awareness of Ki.

No one can tell you what you should experience – for each individual this is unique. Energetic experiences are often not comparable and, as mentioned earlier, are subjective.

This is the beginning of your journey to a new perspective on life.

Earth Ki

About 3 inches (8 cm) below the navel is the symbolic energetic center for Earth Ki, the *hara*. Building Earth Ki creates a solid foundation from which to progress in Japanese energetic teachings. It is imperative that a solid energetic base exists. To understand its importance, imagine the human body as an energetic triangle, with the base of the triangle playing the supporting role.

The *hara* contains one's original

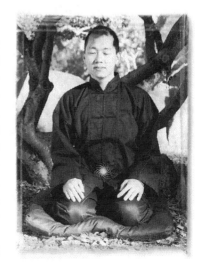

energy. Original energy is the Ki that you are born into this world with. It is not a stagnant energy but something that can be built upon to create this necessary solid foundation. This area of the body is often compared to a wok where cooking takes place. The essential ingredients are added and built upon, one-by-one: sesame oil, ginger, soy sauce, garlic. They are heated and mixed and become the base for the most aromatic and delicious food that one can eat. This is the function of the *hara* to offer a practitioner the foundation from which to develop Ki.

The Ki that emanates from the Earth is heavy, powerful and grounding. This grounding force offers both physical and mental strength. The term 'grounding' generally indicates that a practitioner interacts in a realistic and practical manner with life. To be grounded is to feel strong, secure and safe as well as physically connected to the environment.

Working on one's Earth energy connection develops focus and perseverance and stabilizes the mind. Feet become firmly planted on the Earth in a secure and stable stance. This confidence and practicality is reflected in a practitioner's dealings with the world. Developing the Earth Ki connection helps practitioners deal with emotions such as fear, uncertainty and low self-esteem. This Ki will support and ground stressed or weak practitioners. Solid grounding work with Earth Ki minimizes the possibility of cracks appearing in the foundation during the later stages of practice.

Sensing Earth Ki Technique

This straightforward technique moves energy, developing and supporting awareness of the Earth-human link.

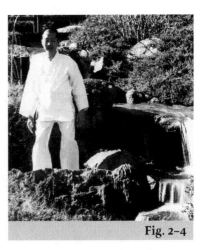

Fig. 2-4

> Stand in a relaxed, yet conscious, manner with your feet spaced hip width apart (Fig. 2–4). Focus your awareness on the centre of the Earth. Experience the pull of the cool, powerful

planet. Your body sinks into it without any physical movement actually occurring. Visualize the center of the Earth in front of you. Intuitively connect to it through your *hara*.

Breathe slowly and regularly. On the in breath feel the energy of the center of the Earth entering your *hara*. Retain this connection as you slowly release the breath. Repeat the in and out breath, connecting with this core Earth Ki, nine times.

Can you perceive the strength you have drawn into your body? Is it steadier, more solid and powerful? Take note of your individual sensations.

Heaven Ki

Emanating from the Heavens is a light, expansive energy known as Heaven Ki. Accessing this energy makes practitioners intuitive and sharp. It has a far less physical quality than Earth Ki.

For visualization purposes Heaven Ki is considered to be associated with the head area. This relates to the development of intuition and mental acuity. The clarity of this energy aids the practicing of stillness, within which practitioners remember their spiritual connection.

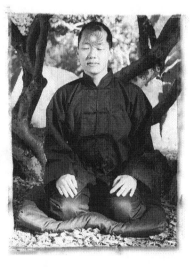

It is also possible when operating in this area that colors or visions are experienced.

Working with Heaven Ki is the next step in the energetic learning process. By beginning at the base, Earth, and then moving to its polar opposite, Heaven, practitioners will avoid problematic imbalances. This method of graduated learning is often ignored today. Many practitioners are taught to work immediately with their Heaven Ki connection, disregarding the importance of their Earth Ki connection. Too often these practitioners end up with their heads in the clouds. For example, an excellent psychic who is not grounded may have a great deal of ability when working with others, but be incapable of solving his or her own issues. This is not deliberate in modern systems but is due to an ignorance of the basic tenets of the system of Reiki.

When you are connected with this centre you may see colors or you might have psychic ability. It is important for you not to become unbalanced, you must keep yourself very centred and grounded. If you can use this energy in a balanced way, you can see beyond the immediate. It is very beautiful but keep things in perspective and do not get carried away with it.

Sensing Heaven Ki Technique

Stand once again in a relaxed, conscious manner with your feet hip width apart (Fig. 2–5). Visualize a ball of bright energy above your head (Fig. 2–6). This beautiful ball draws on the energy from the Heavens.

On the in breath feel this Heavenly ball moving down through your crown, into your heart and finally down to the *hara* (Fig. 2–7).

On the out breath draw the ball back up from the *hara* to your heart and out through the crown until it rests above your head.

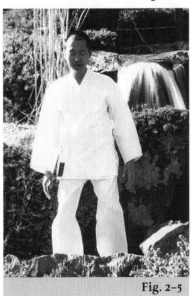

Fig. 2–5

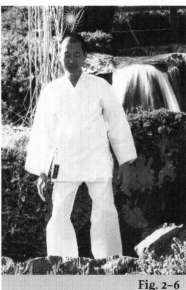

Fig. 2–6

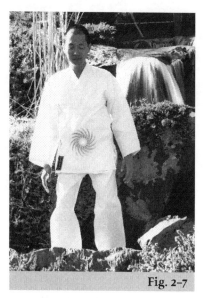

Keep your connection with this ball of Heavenly energy and repeat the breathing and the accompanying visualization nine times.

Are you feeling light and airy, with a certain bright-eyed knowledge about the world? Take your personal knowledge about Heaven Ki and store it in your treasure chest of energetic data.

Fig. 2-7

Heart Ki

The third diamond, Heart Ki, is the point of perfect balance that is created by the merging of Earth and Heaven, body and mind. Heart Ki is symbolically located in the center of the chest. By tapping into Heart energy a practitioner begins to shine, radiating light to all directions. Hurt, pain, resentment, mental trauma, stress, anger and fear are all resolved in this light, inviting more forgiveness, love, peace and compassion into a

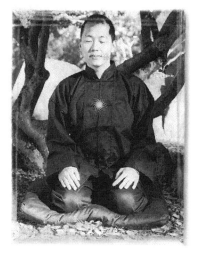

practitioner's life. The polishing of this diamond is in fact the polishing of the self and is the culmination of balancing the mind and body.

Once practitioners achieve this balance their focus moves to the big picture, rather than immediate problems. Issues are dealt with easily and energy is not wasted on worry or fear.

Ueshiba Morihei, founder of *aikidô*, wrote, 'Blend the Heaven and Earth energy with that of your own, becoming life itself. As you calm down, naturally let yourself settle down in the hidden realm of the formless, returning to the heart of things.'

'Returning to the heart of things' is the point of balance reached by harmonizing the body, mind and heart, forming the one perfect diamond – you.

Sensing Heart Ki Technique

In your relaxed, aware stance open your arms and hold them at heart level out from your body as if you are embracing a large tree trunk (Fig. 2–8).

Reach down with your arms and gently gather up the energy of the Earth (Fig. 2–9). Bring it up and into the heart area of your body.

Open your arms again and reach up to Heaven, gathering the Heavenly energy (Fig. 2–10) and bringing it downward and in until your hands are again in front of your heart.

Repeat these movements nine times.

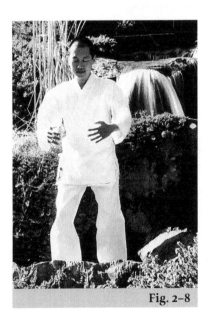
Fig. 2–8

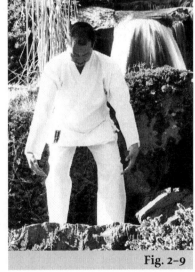
Fig. 2–9

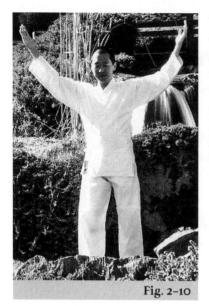

The experience, even fleeting, of this sense of balance may be accompanied by a renewed vigor for 'really living'. You begin to understand that the human experience is not separate from Ki – it is a part of this energy, and life extends beyond our physical boundaries.

Fig. 2–10

Ki Movement

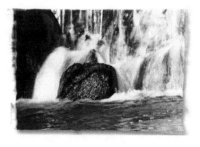

The concept of body, mind and heart can be replicated outside of the human body too. It is an energetic expression of human-kind in general and of the Earth, the universe, even existence. For humans to attain an understanding of the movement of Ki and its irreplaceable function in the world it can be valuable to look at life in these terms. Aim to touch the physical form, know the mind and feel the heart of all things to fully comprehend existence.

Now that it is understood how the energetic body works it is vital to recognize how the system of Reiki utilizes it. The system teaches practitioners techniques to cultivate greater amounts of Ki, or Reiki, with the aim of moving Ki to cleanse and clear the baggage that one takes on board. Practitioners may also place their hands on or just off the body to channel Ki to heal.

By practicing the techniques taught in this system, Earth Ki and Heaven Ki become strong and balanced, and their connection accordingly stimulates powerful Heart Ki. Working directly with the three diamonds cultivates the natural flow of Ki paralleling the aims of the system of Reiki. Ki is constantly moving through the body. The ultimate aim of the system is to create a free flow of energy allowing humans to experience a permanent connection to the universal flow of Ki.

In modern times, Reiki is often thought of solely as a palm-healing technique, with little attention placed on the origin or meaning of the skill. Though humans are born with the ability to channel energy for healing, to develop this skill *successfully* large amounts of energy need to be generated in the body. During a Reiki course a student receives an attunement or *reiju* from the teacher initiating a shift in the student's energy. This shift is a clearing of energy: freeing the flow of energy through the body aiding the cultivation of personal Ki. Simultaneously the student begins to purposefully move Ki in the body during meditation and the practicing of techniques. Together, the student and teacher are laying the foundations for a lifetime practice. There are countless energetic shifts throughout one's life. Practicing this system helps to move through them swiftly, clearing energy that may otherwise have remained stagnant.

3 The Effect of Reiki

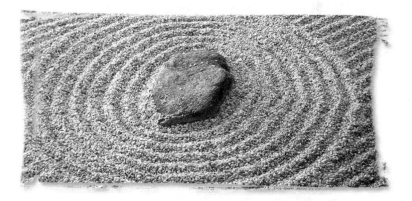

People naturally want to know what the direct effect of working with Reiki will be. Can it help a sore back, cure depression or even rid one of a recurring nightmare? The answer to each of these questions is, 'It may'. Reiki is clearly beneficial, but it is not possible to predict exactly what it will do, where it will go and how it will cure. This is not because Reiki is limited, but rather because humans are too likely to limit Reiki with rational and logical thought processes. Reiki encompasses so much more than that.

To understand the effect of Reiki it must first be perceived that humans are more than physical body alone. There are other essential ingredients in the human make-up including the mind and heart connection. Each of these influences the other – not one is isolated.

A typical example of the mysterious interconnectedness of these elements can be seen in the following imaginary life story of Sato Yoshiko as she comes into contact with the system of Reiki.

The Tale of Sato

For Sato Yoshiko, every day had a sameness about it. She would get up, prepare the family's *bento* or lunch boxes, have breakfast with her husband and their two daughters, walk the girls to primary school and then head to the Tôkyô subway. Here she would stand with the other commuters on the platform, allowing herself to be squeezed into the train carriage. She would be squashed on every side of her body until she no longer felt her own physical boundaries. She would close her eyes and imagine she was anywhere but on that train.

Once at her destination, the Ginza district, she flowed with the crowds arriving at the Mitsukoshi Department store, her workplace. Downstairs in the food hall she donned her uniform and served customers with traditional Japanese sweets. By early afternoon she was worn out and was constantly struggling to remain friendly and kind to her customers and colleagues. Her feet began to ache and her arthritic knee pained her.

Sato's day finished in much the same way it had begun. She returned by train to pick up her daughters, preparing and eating dinner with her family and finally falling into bed before beginning again the next day.

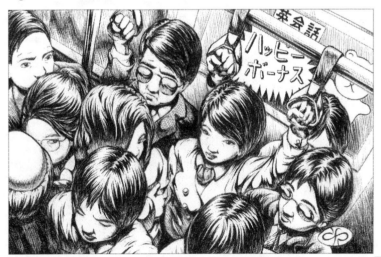

Sato's father died when he was only sixty and she was devastated. He had always been there for her whenever there had been indecision or difficulties in her life. Her mother, too, had relied greatly on her father and was finding his transition extremely hard to comprehend. Sato tried to support her, being the only child, but found that she did not have the inner strength to deal with both her mother's and her own grief. Sato's family and colleagues began to notice that all was not well. She no longer laughed or spoke much. Everyone felt she had closed up and was 'inside of herself'. The doctor diagnosed her as depressed. He prescribed tablets for her but she refused to take them as she was worried they might not be good for her. Her family was uncertain what to do or where to go next.

A colleague of her husband suggested that she go for a Reiki treatment at a local Reiki center. Not knowing what this Reiki was, Sato hesitantly agreed and arrived for the treatment nervous but hopeful.

Her practitioner first talked to her about the treatment. She explained that Sato would be lying down for the treatment but did not need to remove any clothes. The practitioner also set Sato's mind at ease by stating that she would not be placing her hands on any private parts of her body and may not even touch her physically.

Sato learnt that all she had to do was relax and feel 'open' for healing to occur, and it would then be up to her whether or not that healing took place. The practitioner was simply a channel for the Ki to move through and Sato's body would draw on it where it needed and wanted it. Sato felt good about this as it meant that she was not relying on the practitioner to make her better – her own strength would do that. She had always felt that no one could understand her unique problems. This concept of healing as a self-responsibility weighed on her but also showed her a doorway that she sensed could lead to recovery along a natural path. This 'Reiki' felt right.

The practitioner told Sato at her first treatment: 'Reiki is not diagnostic. My hands on your body immediately activate the movement of energy. Therefore Ki is already working away at healing and cleansing your body. Diagnosing with Reiki would merely be pandering to the practitioner's need for control or power. The real challenge is not to understand what is energetically happening but how NOT to understand. Learning to let go is beneficial to every aspect of life.'

The Ki, her practitioner further explained, would wash down through her energetic pathways clearing stagnant energy. This movement of Ki would initiate change for Sato but the practitioner could not foretell what that change might be. This would depend on what Sato needed right now. Her practitioner stressed that she could not make any claims to achieve specific results for Sato – it was a matter of letting go for both of them and seeing what the result would be.

The practitioner also asked why she was here and Sato quietly answered that she had been diagnosed as depressed. Sato learnt that even if she was taking prescription medicine, it would still be safe to receive a Reiki treatment.

Sensing Sato's insecurity about the system, her practitioner explained a little more about safety issues and Reiki. It seemed that the belief that Reiki cannot harm is based on the understanding that the system works without deliberately manipulating Ki. Manipulation, Sato was assured, is a human habit not a universal one. Therefore any danger comes not through tapping into the source and drawing more Ki through the body. This relates to balance, and balance only. Of course, said Sato's practitioner, it is humans themselves that can be dangerous. They can say things that are inappropriate or act in a way that creates an unsafe environment for others. Therefore practitioners of the system of Reiki working professionally must be experienced and should be able to be held accountable either through an association or established organization. Any risk linked with the system of Reiki is human rather than energetic. Her practitioner at the same time indicated her practice where her own certificates, codes of practice and ethics and association membership were hanging.

Sato lay on the futon with her eyes open for the first five

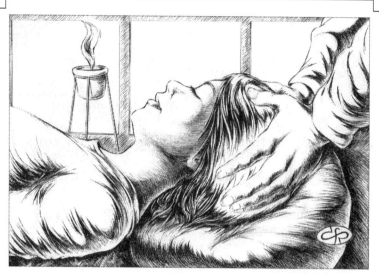

minutes or so, even though she had been told it was okay to close them. She just could not relax. The practitioner began at her head and moved down the front of her body. Sato could feel hands on her body and, interestingly, she could even feel it when they were just off her body too. She felt some sort of static energy running through her scalp and hair and then a sensation of heat over her eyes. Suddenly something in her got very heavy. She gave a loud, unrestrained sigh and her shoulders dropped, her eyes closed and she softly began to snore. Funnily enough, even though to an observer it appeared she was fast asleep she was totally aware of what was going on around her. It was as if her physical body had said that it had had enough and wanted to sleep but her mind, and something else that she couldn't quite put her finger on, were active. Startling, sharp images flashed through her mind impressing pictures on the insides of her eyes. Each image had a symbolic relevance that she instantly comprehended but when the treatment finished after an hour she could remember very little about them.

A few minutes later the practitioner offered her a glass of water – to help the cleansing process she was told. Sato related her experience and went on to say that at certain hand positions she also felt waves of energy moving down through her arms and legs. All of these experiences were supposedly quite common and some people felt the same sensations on different parts of the body. These sensations indicated quite clearly that something had occurred but Sato had no idea what. The practitioner very simply told her that it was a good sign that she could feel so much and she was sure that the treatment would be beneficial for Sato in whatever way her body desired it to be so.

Sato was stunned that she had been able to relax so quickly. Snoring might not be the most charming way to relax but it did indicate an easing of tension and stress. The nights of lying in bed with her eyes staring at nothingness in the dark had started her thinking that she would never be able to sleep with ease again. If she learnt to work on herself with Ki, perhaps she would be able to sleep this well all by herself.

'Well, what should I do next?' Sato enquired.

She could have another two treatments if she felt that the treatments would continue to be helpful. Ultimately though, she was told, learning to practice Reiki on herself would be far more powerful. This was true for many reasons, as she would one day find out.

Within two weeks, feeling brave and suddenly eager about this new challenge in her life, Sato found herself sitting in a small class of people with her practitioner now in the role of teacher. Three other women and two men were in her class. Each looked to be of a different age and economic background. Their reasons for joining the Reiki course differed – some believed that they had healing hands; others had sick family members they wanted to help. One older woman said that she, just like Sato, was studying it to help herself. The teacher told them all that they must first focus on healing themselves, as this was the most important aspect of the system of Reiki.

The course was very practical. Sato first learnt about meditation. This was something she had always been curious about but had related it to religious or New Age groups. However, she did have an uncle who swore by the benefits of it. She followed directions and soon she was effortlessly feeling the movement of Ki in her body. She got so hot she thought she might have to stop but the practice itself finished first.

As someone new to the system of Reiki, the time spent concentrating on what was happening energetically in her body allowed Sato to feel things she may never have been aware of – actual physical sensations of Ki such as tingling, heat and rushes of energy. This was the physical proof that she needed to open herself up even further to experience energetic growth.

It seemed that the more that she practiced moving Ki the faster that change would occur and that was fine with her. But it also meant practice, practice, practice. At this point she was not quite sure what changes would occur but she was enjoying these new sensations enough to trust that it would be to her benefit.

A cathartic realization that humans are energetic and spiritual beings lifted her out of the mundaneness of life. It offered form to a world that she had no longer felt able to deal with – it offered hope. This 'physical' experience of energy was like a reminder of a connection, though perhaps tenuous at first, with 'home'.

Listening to everyone's insights she was amazed how each person described their experiences differently. Some saw lights or even other 'people', experienced heightened sound or smell or other 'new' experiences.

These first encounters indicated that what was once considered normal in everyday life held many new and unforeseen secrets. The students started to think outside of the square.

Initially, Sato found that working consciously with Ki appeared to affect her perceptions. She knew that humans rarely saw themselves as anything but a physically functioning body with a very busy mind.

The simple action of thinking consciously about Ki and its relationship to daily life immediately affected change. To be confronted with the concept that the natural flow of the universe is inside each person, and consequently that the actions of each person affect this flow, Sato found astonishing.

In Sato's manual there was a quote she felt summed up her awe at her newly acquired understanding. It was from Yamada Etai, former head priest of the Tendai sect. He wrote in the foreword of *Right View, Right Life* by Kohno Jiko, 'Among the teachings of the Tendai sect of Japanese Buddhism is one about 'three thousands realms in one mind'. This is the idea that the action of one's mind in a single instant contains 'three thousand realms,' or the entire universe, and therefore if our mind acts it can affect the entire cosmos. Realizing that, we can say that worldliness is giving rise to the environmental problems of acid rain, global warming, rapid depletion of forests, pollution of rivers, lakes and oceans and the desertification of our planet – crises that affect the continued existence of the human race.'

The meditations and her reawakened understanding of the purpose of her three Ki centers were preparing Sato for another inexplicable event.

All of the students were asked to sit to receive *reiju*. Each student sat as this ritual was performed by the teacher. It took only a couple of minutes, leaving the student to sit quietly in the energy for a while longer.

This blessing by the teacher brought to Sato something that was not physical or a matter of changed perception. If her link to that inner 'home' had been tenuous half an hour ago, suddenly it was potent. When asked about her experience with the *reiju* she looked at the faces of those in her group and excused herself saying, 'I can't explain how I feel but something important has happened.' Later that day she tried to explain it to her family as they sat around listening to her Reiki adventures. She told them she had made direct contact with something unique in herself and this was all before lunchtime! But, she told them, she had been lucky because not everyone felt what she had and some just said that their impression of the *reiju* was one of peace. This mysterious *reiju* was explained as a technique that the teacher performed to create a space in which Sato's healing and sense of connectedness could safely take place.

'The *reiju* coupled with meditation and techniques,' the teacher explained, 'will allow greater amounts of Ki to flow through you. This will improve your mind and body and enable you to purposefully channel energy for healing through the palms, eyes and breath.'

When it was time for Sato to receive a full treatment on the first day of the course she felt comforted knowing what lay in store. She was to receive a one-hour treatment from the older woman, the one who had stated her wish to also work on herself. This woman appeared a little nervous as she was being thrown in the deep end. Her teacher assured them all that being able to immediately work with Reiki only accentuated the simplicity of the palm-healing aspect of the system. They were then taught that a practitioner need only hold one clear intention in the mind. This intention must always be that the client, in this case Sato, may receive whatever she needed at this particular moment in time. A practitioner does not manipulate or stimulate the energy but becomes an open vessel for Ki to flow through. The more open and the stronger a practitioner becomes by practicing the meditations the more energy can flow through her or him.

The treatment commenced and Sato's eyes closed immediately. Once again, she began to gently snore her way through the next hour.

'What was that in my knee?' she exclaimed, sitting up after the treatment.

She felt totally invigorated this time though during the treatment she had had pains shooting through her right knee as well as shaking. Both Sato and the woman looked at each other wide eyed and laughed. Not only did Sato think she had found a key to open a new experience in her life but also, perhaps, a new friend. To her utter amazement even her knee felt less arthritic as she gingerly stood up. Her friend was more skeptical. She had not really felt much (except for the shaking knee!) and did not seem convinced she could really do it even though Sato kept reassuring her how great it had been.

After listening to the class's experiences with their first treatment, their teacher said: 'Sometimes pain, illness, even shaking or welling up of emotions is felt during or after Ki work.

On the other hand you may also become extremely happy or re-energized. Everything that occurs is considered a cleansing. It is the Ki moving things inside you, creating change. This may not always be entirely pleasant but it is effective. The more open that a practitioner is to change the greater the change that occurs. There are less obstructions and the movement can occur with ease. No one ever knows what this movement will be but it is accepted that it will always be for the benefit of the practitioner. Please know that these occurrences are not considered 'good' or 'bad' – they simply are. And once we move through them we enter a new plateau where balance is created in our life. Each of you is here because you want change in your lives and here it is.'

On the morning of the second day the students discussed how their own meditation and palm-healing had been during their home practice. When it was Sato's turn the class looked at her strangely. Sato later questioned her friend who told her that Sato's face had altered. The shadow that her features seemed to cast yesterday appeared gone. She looked lighter. Sato admitted to feeling lighter too. She did not feel as weighed down as she had over the past few months and there had been a renewed freshness in her step this morning as she walked to the center.

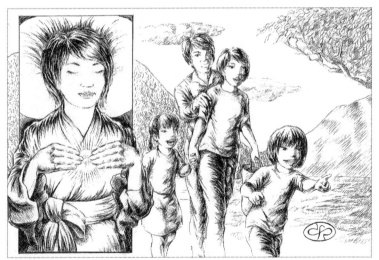

Something that inspired Sato was the creed of Usui. This consists of five precepts: profound thoughts created to bring our mind into the awareness of our present state.

By the end of her second day she had a glimmer of the possible changes she could make to her life and the benefits she would reap. She would create a daily routine of meditation and palm-healing with the incorporation of the Usui creed. Her aim would be to touch and cultivate her inner strength and spiritual connection. To support her conviction to create change she would also attend a weekly practice group with her teacher, practicing techniques and palm healing in a group environment.

Sato's family was amazed at her turn around. She truly had found a new light within herself. Her change of attitude affected everyone. Hope and enjoyment in life had made her a pleasure to be around. Friends who had recently been concerned and quiet around her opened up and shared in her enthusiasm. Her husband almost felt shy in her light.

'You may think that it is strange that I can feel so different, so suddenly,' Sato declared to her husband, 'but I am looking with new eyes at my old world.'

After a month or two, Sato's husband asked carefully if she believed that she would always retain her new perceptions and healing abilities or would they fade away? Sato had initially wondered this herself and spoke to him about what she now believed. 'Naturally, we can grow lazy and our perceptions can slide back to where we once were. But Ki will never fully disappear as humans are born as energetic beings. We all have that great diamond within us – we just need to continue to polish it. It is the cultivation of this Ki that makes the difference. I must continue to do this to maintain my spiritual growth. I will continue to practice on myself with meditations and palm-healing and subsequently receive all these wonderful benefits that I now enjoy.'

Sato went on to list what she knew to be different in her life. Due to her strong commitment she had moved on from depression and found a stronger core inside herself. She knew that core could be much stronger still but it was already beginning to sustain her as a balanced and content human.

Physically, she felt strong and her knee had not irritated her since she had completed the course. At work she felt robust and did not tire quite as easily. Whether this was from an improved attitude toward her work or from a sturdier inner energy, or both, she did not know and neither did it matter, she thought. Her colleagues had all commented on what a joy it was to work with her and customers smiled when they saw her coming. These reactions spurred her on to maintain her practice and so everything continued to develop. Sato thought about how her smiling customers felt affected by her warm light. She believed that they could not help but be kinder to the next salesperson they dealt with that day who, in turn, would feel pleased to be treated so respectfully and give that little bit more in their next exchange and so on.

At home Sato found herself attracted to other new interests. Even her husband's and daughters' *bento* boxes received the once-over after she read some interesting books about the benefits of eating organic food that was not genetically modified. The inevitable daily Tôkyô subway experience was replaced with a bike ride and Sato's lunchtime no longer took place while window-shopping but on a bench overlooking a duck-filled pond in the Ginza's Hibiya-kôen park.

The physical experience of working with Ki that she had felt during the course eventually become less sporadic. The heightened sense of Ki movement became a normal state as she regularly practiced. Her experience taught her that these sensations can be viewed as a side effect of her journey but must never be confused with the journey itself. Some of her weekly practice group had feared that heightened senses might be an issue for them in daily life but this was never the case.

One group regular expressed his thoughts on this: 'To be aware of energetic change is not the same as being buffeted by it. Walking into a room where there has been an argument definitely does not mean that you become argumentative or upset. What it can lead to is an awareness that may well be useful when dealing with the room's participants. The more that the practitioner works on the self the more balance and understanding the practitioner achieves. This stability and groundedness goes hand in hand with heightened experience.'

Others who had completed the course with her kept in contact through the weekly practice group. Some had great personal growth and some had setbacks but most had a bit of both. After six months, two no longer went to the weekly group and she knew that their interest in self-development had waned. Her friend, who had not had Sato's initial revelatory experience, grew gradually more confident in her practice to become a solid practitioner – her understanding was deep and the two had many supportive and fruitful conversations together about the profundity of Ki work.

Through everything, Sato knew that the most important aspect of what she had learnt was for her to grow as a spiritual being and from this point she could naturally affect all whom she met along her path.

In time she knew she would study the second level of the system of Reiki to learn about the symbols and mantras associated with it, discovering new methods to develop her understanding. Then, perhaps one day, she might even continue on to become what is called a Reiki teacher or master, a teacher of the system. Though she may well accept the title, she knew to become a master of something so omnipresent and great would most likely remain a task 'under construction'.

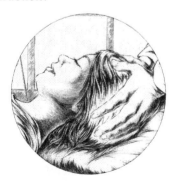

Healing

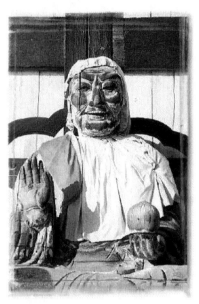

The word 'heal' has many different interpretations. To clearly describe 'heal' the definition 'to make whole' is often used. 'To make whole' means to balance out all aspects of being human: the body, mind and heart. It embraces the concept of the interconnectedness of these aspects and does not accept that one is of more import than another.

Does conventional Western medicine therefore make a person whole? An aspirin or panadol will mask a problem – not heal it. An operation will remove or reconfigure something so that it functions better but does not heal the original cause or the consequent trauma associated with surgery. Conventional Western medicine excels technically at many levels but has become an unbalanced treatment unable 'to make whole' humankind. The health industry is supported by governmental systems that appear more interested in reaping the benefits from pharmaceutical companies than supporting the growth of happy, healthy citizens. This current structure does not take seriously the need for individuals to feel emotional fulfillment, to believe that there is meaning to their lives or to discover their spiritual connection.

Healing humanity, making whole, affects the individual and therefore naturally heals the greater society too. Healing should result in lowering suicide rates, removing war, criminality and discontentment in general. The idea of an innate sense of contentment is foreign to most of humankind and this lack can be viewed as the root of many of the world's troubles. Conventional Western medicine does not touch these issues and appears more focused on what we might call 'longevity': extending our physical experience of life – but what use is longevity if life is hell? Even in dying, a natural phase for the physical human body, there can be wholeness.

The ancients did not consider longevity to be a striving toward an extended lifetime, as we do today. Longevity represented the attaining of a spiritual connection: to 'become One' or perhaps to 'make whole'. Withered or dead, they realized that their physical bodies were inconsequential. They knew that the experience of becoming One with the universe meant that there was in fact no beginning or end.

Nowadays there is a lack of spiritual connection due to a fear of the unknown; namely death. Instead of strengthening a spiritual connection and developing the concept of whole beings that can deal with these mystical issues, modern people simply hold onto life for as long as they can. This desperation means a constant fighting against death, leaving little time or energy to look at aspects of what it might mean to live life well and in the Now.

In China, traditionally each village had a doctor. This doctor was charged with keeping all villagers well and healthy. As long as this was accomplished the doctor would be paid a regular stipend but once there was sickness – payment was withheld. The culture believed that the doctor did not deserve to be paid for poor work. Perhaps the doctor had not noticed that a specific Qi Gong technique was no longer suitable for a villager or that a stored food crop was too old and no longer nutritious. The doctor's responsibility was to keep an eye on the holistic elements of the villagers' lives and guide them where necessary.

In Japan, historically the spiritual practitioners performed healing. The spiritual guidance and practices that took place might be considered as superstitious nonsense by modern society. They used forms of divination, mediumship and meditation; yet, at the same time these beliefs and rituals were protection for the clans.

The contrast here with what occurs today is that the focus was on maintaining healthy lives and prevention of illness. Due to a lack of connection today life is lived until it is about to fall apart and then there is a frantic race against time to patch it back together again. Humanity is currently not in the process of healing but is receiving a bandage over a wound that cannot heal without the correct care.

Presently, how to find this correct care is of the essence to everyone. There are many avenues one can take and it is for the individual to decide which road is best suited to his or her needs. The system of

Reiki attempts to make humanity whole by using five elements that, when joined together, create a unique and deeply effective method.

Sato Yoshiko was not completely healed. She realized that her human task was to heal the wound inside herself and to do this embarked on what might be called 'her healing journey'. Whether humanity is aware of it or not, there is a healing journey for everyone to take and the choice is whether to actively embrace it or not.

This is the ultimate responsibility – to care for oneself and work toward the creation of a whole person. It cannot be achieved by anyone else. As with the Chinese doctor, guidance is invaluable but the effort that reaps results can only come from the self. A spiritual road is allotted to everyone and it is up to the individual as to how far, if at all, that is traveled.

It is wise to remember that humanity has put the systems in place that govern its people. This includes the daily menial structures as well as a country's greater administrative bodies. Society cannot acknowledge spirituality on a greater scale if the people do not discover it for themselves. How one life is lived affects the world.

Ensure that your life is an effective one.

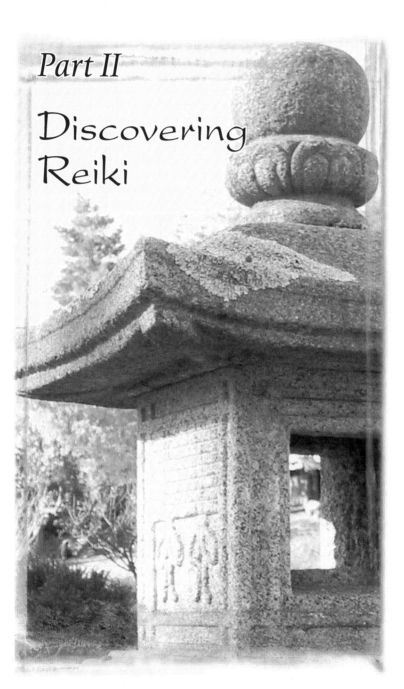

Part II

Discovering Reiki

4 The Five Elements

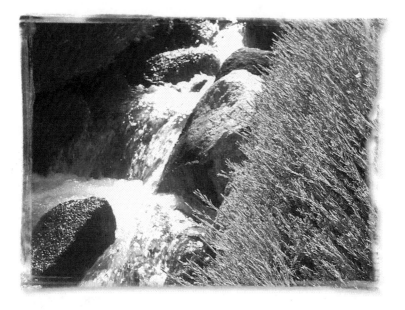

All five elements of the system of Reiki are reliant upon one another to ensure an effective, complete system. To define the exact nature of each element their characteristics have been divided up into sections. This layout offers the reader a quick and easy reference guide to all aspects of the five elements.

The sections for each element are:

Description: The element is fully described: clarifying its function within the system and at what level it is taught.

Source: The origin and general background of the element is discussed for an integrated understanding of the system's roots.

Rewards: The benefits of working with the element are revealed.

Application: The practical application of how to use the element is taught.

Questions: By answering these questions a deeper and more personal understanding of each element, and your relationship to it, is attained.

Description

Throughout the system of Reiki's global trotting and time traveling, just five elements have remained consistent. Many other aspects have been removed, altered or created over the last hundred years. Culturally, the system has adapted itself to various traditions where it has been modified to suit the moral and spiritual values unique to each tradition. Individually, it has also been molded to the tastes and skills of practitioners – and yet these five basic elements have remained. Often in the past, this survival has been reliant on unusual guises that reflect, once again, a cultural or individual influence. Therefore it is easy to understand why for many practitioners today it is a challenge to see the system's five elements clearly.

To bring the system back to an essential core by working through each of these elements from a self-practice viewpoint is the aim of Part II of *The Japanese Art of Reiki*. Here can be discovered, or rediscovered, by practical means the distinctiveness of the system's beauty and power.

It has already been described how the basis of the system was created by a Japanese man, Usui Mikao, in the early 1900s from his own unique experiences. Usui's blending of esoteric Buddhism called Mikkyô, ancient Shugendô practices, classical *samurai* teachings, and martial arts know-how produced distinctive teachings. By utilizing traditional approaches in his own inimitable way his intention was to bring about an unmasking, a revelation of what it meant to be human.

Consequently, it is not the energy itself that makes this system unique but the path that is walked. This path developed into one consisting of five elements: *gokai* (daily precepts), *kokyû hô* (breathing techniques), *tenohira* (palm-healing), *shirushi* and *jumon* (symbols and mantras), and the receiving of *reiju* from a teacher (a blessing from which the Western attunement evolved).

A practitioner practices the majority of these elements alone – *gokai, kokyû hô,* and *shirushi* and *jumon. Tenohira,* too, is practiced on oneself with the possibility of using it on others. These elements all become part of a personal daily routine coupled with the regular receiving of *reiju* from a teacher where possible. When brought together each of the elements exerts a separate influence on the practitioner producing a complete system that affects powerful change.

Source

Those that knew Usui tell of a humble man, one who did not even see himself as a teacher. Teachers of the system of Reiki can learn much about the system from this information. An idea has grown in the West that teachers are in control of a student's ability to draw on Ki by bestowing a 'magical gift' (called a *reiju* or more recently an attunement) on the student. These teachers also believe they have the ability to withdraw, alter or even negate Ki.

For two reasons this is inaccurate if viewed from a traditional perspective. It undermines the concept of Reiki as the energy of everything – energy with an ultimate, innate knowledge that is outside of human comprehension. It also takes away from the basic premise that working with the system develops a practitioner's self-responsibility – only you can heal yourself. To rely on a teacher to receive personal growth and healing will surely end in poor long-term results. Students lose the majority of their received 'power' (or at least their belief in it) often returning to their teacher for a 'fix' as this magic no longer seems to work. This is due to the teacher being seen as the 'powerful' figure in the teacher/student relationship and can easily become a profitable and unethical system. The other important issue is that as this structure creates teachers who believe they are more powerful than the student, ego driven teaching is being generated. Fortunately, this concept is becoming outdated as students (and teachers) grow to become more educated with the importance of self-practice being acknowledged. In this case, knowledge IS power: self-power.

Ongoing individual work evidences great change for a practitioner. This is where the path of dedicated work leads. To understand this more fully it is helpful to follow the path of Usui. Usui did not receive the understanding of his teachings within a short period of time: he had to work hard by practicing meditations, copying sutras (texts), undertaking mountain retreats and much more. It is stated on the Usui memorial stone that two thousand students completed *Shoden* (Level I), and of this just sixty to seventy went on to *Okuden* (Level II) and of those approximately only twenty became *Shinpiden* (Level III). If the system was so easy and based solely on receiving *reiju* with little or no emphasis on personal practice then more people would have moved through to the higher levels.

Rewards

Using each of these five elements individually is a strong practice yet when you combine them they produce a complete spiritual teaching that is accessible to everyone. Each element supports the other, filling in the gaps that will exist for different practitioners. No two people have the same needs when learning. For this reason working with all five elements gives each practitioner a greater chance of success. Together these elements create a whole that is firm yet flexible, supporting practitioners on their individual spiritual paths.

If practitioners tread in the footsteps of Usui (metaphorically) with steadfast self-practice they will be assured of discovering deeper, more consistent and lasting results from the system of Reiki.

Application

The five elements appear at different levels of the system of Reiki. Some are repeated as a part of all three levels in varied forms while the importance of others is restricted to just the one level. For clarity, a table is provided that associates the five elements and their uses with specific levels of the system (Fig. 4–1).

Level	Purpose	Five Elements
Shoden **Level I**	To learn to sense Ki, cultivate Ki and use this knowledge to ground and heal the self (healing others for non-professional use may also be taught).	*Gokai* – Develop the spiritual and mental connection using *gokai* (five precepts). ***Kokyû hô*** – Learn *kokyû hô* (breathing techniques) appropriate to this level to ground the student. ***Tenohira*** –The physical practice of *tenohira* (palm-healing) on the self/others for the purpose of healing. ***Reiju*** – Receive *reiju* (a blessing) from a teacher to develop the student's energetic connection.
Okuden **Level II**	To learn extra tools to strengthen a practitioner's knowledge and connection with Ki. Using Ki to connect to others not within physical reach for healing (healing others for professional use may also be taught).	***Kokyû hô*** – Learn *kokyû hô* appropriate to this level to generate more energy. ***Jumon*** and ***Shirushi*** – Learn three *jumon* and three *shirushi* to aid the student in focusing Ki and 'becoming' the appropriate energies. ***Reiju*** – Receive *reiju* from a teacher to develop the student's energetic connection.
Shinpiden **Level III** (Also known as Reiki teacher, Reiki master or 3a and 3b in the West)	To focus on furthering personal development and the passing of the system of Reiki on to others.	***Kokyû hô*** – Learn *kokyû hô* appropriate to this level to advance deeper into personal spirituality. ***Jumon*** and ***Shirushi*** – Learn one *jumon* and one *shirushi* to aid the student in focusing Ki and 'becoming' the appropriate energy. ***Reiju*** – Receive *reiju* and learn how to perform *reiju* on others.

Fig. 4-1   The Five Elements

Within a Reiki course there will undoubtedly be other elements included that are integral to offering a professional and thorough learning experience. The teacher's interests, culture and Ki background generally dictate these. It will also depend on the length and structure of the course (how many days, or weeks, or is it the duration of a lifetime?) the legal responsibilities for practitioners in some countries, and other variables.

Before beginning with the practices in this book it is wise to have an understanding of how to prepare yourself. To prepare for any practice in the system of Reiki a number of observances are followed. Some of these are conscious while others occur naturally and are relatively unconscious.

After much practice, preparations may become second nature though it is always most beneficial to keep your awareness in the present moment of your practice. Know what it is you are doing, and you will experience a constant sense of aliveness. Your practice will then be lifted from an inconvenient task to an enjoyable aspect of your regular daily experience.

These preparations may also be viewed as rituals. Ritual is integral to the development of one's practice. It offers guidelines to work from, helping a practitioner to direct intention with ease. If one is unsure how to sit or stand or where to place the eyes then each moment spent wondering about these preparations is a distraction: one that draws the intention away, creating a less successful practice.

Even in one's daily life, clarity of intention is what decides whether an action is successful or not: be it a job interview, making a cake, telling a story, driving a car safely or just shopping. Taking a wrong turn in the car or confusing cake ingredients is due to a lack of attention to the job at hand. Humans need to know what it is they are going to do and how they are going to do it to accomplish their aims. This is a reminder of the importance of being present in this very moment of life.

It is at the very beginning of your journey that ritual is integral. The set up that it creates in your mind and body before practicing is essential to achieving your ends. Initially, you may find the practice itself to be difficult to concentrate on or to learn, so to know that you are doing it correctly in a manner that supports the practice is immeasurably beneficial. Once you become more comfortable with your practice you will see that the ritual you have followed has assisted you by setting you in the right frame of mind and correct body position. This will then become second nature within your practice and eventually integrate itself into your daily life.

Basic principles apply prior to beginning a practice. These principles are the ritualized forms that will support you in your practice.

The Six Principles

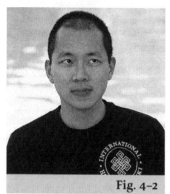
Fig. 4–2

1. First decide which practice you are about to begin (Fig. 4–2). Is it a specific meditation or technique, palm-healing or *reiju*? The decision making process itself kick-starts the practice. Practitioners are often amazed that they feel the flow of energy *prior* to their actual practices. Some receive shocks of energy through their bodies just reading about the workings of Reiki. Connection and intention immediately sharpen as you ready yourself to start.

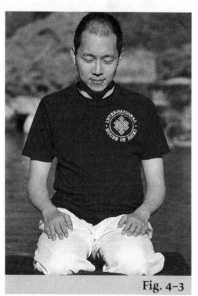
Fig. 4–3

2. Depending upon the practice you will either sit or stand and occasionally lie. To sit for Japanese techniques you should sit in *seiza* (Fig. 4–3). If this is too uncomfortable, sitting in an erect position on a chair is also acceptable. *Seiza*, or correct sitting, is a traditional Japanese style of sitting back on the ankles, with the legs folded underneath and the back erect. Traditionally the process

of sitting in *seiza* is very exact and proceeds with total awareness in a smooth, slow and methodical manner.

Have you ever seen children in pre-school sitting on the floor at story time? Their backs are straight, their hearts are open, their eyes are intensely focused on their teacher and their minds are eager to learn. This is a naturally balanced state. As humans age they begin to cover and defend themselves, taking on physical and emotional baggage to weigh body parts down into all strange shapes and sizes. When walking – they shuffle or skitter, when sitting – they can become shapeless sacks. The truth is that good posture affects human thoughts and vice versa. Once either the thought processes or human posture is corrected change becomes apparent. Not only for themselves but also for those they meet.

The body is in many ways a physical representation of the mind. If a practitioner is sitting in *seiza*, spine curved, shoulders hunched and face screwed up, it is unlikely that this person's mind is at ease. On the other hand if a practitioner is sitting straight, with the chest open – a sense of expansive calm is a natural place for the mind to inhabit. These observances can be carried over into daily life with posture reflecting the inner strengths of a practitioner. Enthusiasm, great spirits and vibrant looks are an inspiration for others. Daily practice reminds practitioners of their natural posture and state of mind. The more this is practiced the more the baggage gets left behind and life is experienced from a connected state.

To sit in *seiza*, bend the legs at the knees with first the right then the left knee being placed on the floor. The left knee is placed about 8 inches (20cm) from the right. Hunch forward over your knees and then settle back to sit onto your ankles with your big toes just touching one another. If the legs tire or fall asleep you can slightly rise up off the knees to allow better circulation or rock back and forth. A pillow or meditation stool can also be placed behind the knees to help lift pressure off the heels. The spine is slightly s-shaped in a naturally stretched position.

Sitting supported by *seiza* releases stress from the body keeping it light and buoyant. Shoulders and arms are relaxed

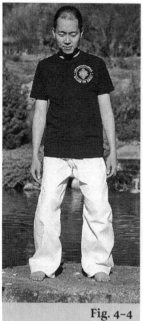

Fig. 4–4

with the palms of the hands facing downward onto the knees.

If you must stand during a practice, the feet are placed hip width apart (Fig. 4–4). The weight of the body is on the toes and the ball of the feet. This stance encourages the upper body's weight to fall naturally to the center called the *hara* (see point 5). Lower the heel back to the ground without placing too much pressure on it. In this position the knees are relaxed and very slightly bent, the shoulders are loose, and the face is calm and relaxed. Arms rest at the sides of the body. There is no tension in the body. This form of relaxation is far stronger than tension. When tense, the body is brittle and can snap but in relaxation there is fluidity and flexibility supporting natural ability.

To lie down during a practice it is preferable not to do so in bed for the simple reason that this is your sleeping area. Bed triggers an accelerated state of relaxation and is likely to put you to sleep rather than support your practice. There is no specific form to lie in as long as the body is relaxed and comfortable. A bolster placed under the knees is advantageous to take the pressure off the lower back when lying flat on the back.

3. The eyes gaze gently at the floor 3 feet (1 meter) in front of the body during meditative exercises (Fig.4-5) or focus straight ahead for more physically directed techniques.

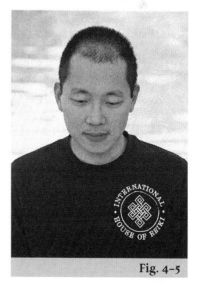

Fig. 4–5

4. Release all tension from your body. Tension only inhibits the free flow of Ki through the body. This does not mean collapsing on the spot but rather experiencing the relaxation of muscles, bones, blood, oxygen and mind, thus enabling the creation of a state of balance across all human levels: be it body, mind or heart.

5. Whether sitting or standing there is a point in the body that must be of major awareness to all practitioners – the *hara* (Fig. 4–6). Described as the body's energetic center for Earth Ki, this is the point of balance that all practitioners acknowledge before beginning their practice. The word *hara* literally means stomach, abdomen or belly. About 3 inches (8 cm) below the navel is where this energy

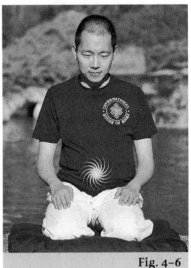

Fig. 4–6

collects with some techniques expanding it out through the entire body. This is a center point of energetic balance for practitioners.

6. You are now ready to begin the actual practice. At this point the hands automatically rise in *gasshô* (Fig. 4–7). This literally means 'to place the two palms together'. These hands are placed in front of the upper body. The higher the hands, the more respect that you are showing. The bringing together of the hands joins both sides of a human, the *in* and *yo* (yin and yang), left and right: creating unity in the one person. Hands are not tense but alive and are held with a small space between the palms.

   The stillness of holding the hands in one position creates a pause and in this moment the mind becomes centered bringing about a state of awareness. Awareness is the foundation for the success of all practices. For one moment be entirely aware of reading this book. Notice how your eyes move across the page, the color of the paper and the shape of the letters, how your body is seated, how your shoulders feel, where your hands are resting, what position your feet are in, where your thighs touch the chair, hear

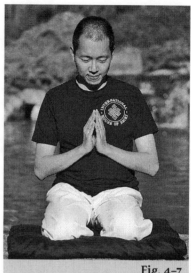

Fig. 4-7

the sounds of the world and smell your surroundings. Notice each thought as it enters and watch where it goes. Be right in this very moment. There is a sense of real living in this instant – that is perfect. This is how you want to experience everything in life. With practice you can gradually make this sensation not a unique event but the experience of everyday living. All traditional Reiki techniques begin and end with *gasshô*. As you will see, some even include *gasshô* as the main practice.

Questions

1. Why do you wish to work on yourself? List your reasons.
2. What excuses do you use to avoid change in your life?
3. Are you ready to begin a practice that may disrupt your regular daily routine? Acknowledge the strengths and weaknesses of your current routine.
4. Can you imagine following through with a practice for longer than 1 week, 1 month, 1 year or longer?

5 Gokai

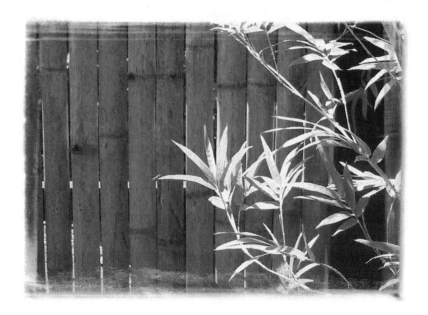

Gokai – five precepts

Description

For today only:
    Do not anger
    Do not worry
    Be humble
    Be honest in your work
    Be compassionate to yourself and others[1]

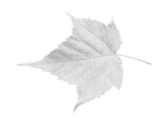

This is a translation of the five precepts as taught in the system of Reiki. A precept is a code of practice. Usui taught them to support his students on their spiritual path of self-healing – they are the baseline to the complete system. These precepts *are* the teachings of Usui, the roots to what has become the system of Reiki. If one were to practice the precepts alone, the spiritual journey would be swift and triumphant. Their deceiving simplicity undercuts the struggle that is relentlessly experienced when working with them. Though the precepts may lie at the heart of the teachings, the enormity of this challenge prompted Usui to create other methods to support practitioners: these are the other four elements of the system of Reiki.

Apart from the five precepts found in the Japanese text, this creed of Usui also includes a brief introduction, directions for use and background information.[2] The creed is in fact a set of fundamental beliefs and directions guiding practitioners on their spiritual journey.

Preceding the five precepts in Usui's creed is an introduction:

> The secret of inviting happiness through many blessings, the spiritual medicine for all illness.

This introduction explains that the 'blessings' of the system are the merit that one receives from practicing the five elements of the system of Reiki. Merit includes all benefits realized by individuals and, as a spin-off, society in general.

Following the five precepts are these practical directions for use:

> Do *gasshô* every morning and evening, keep in your mind and recite.

This is describing the hand position, *gasshô*, which one must hold when reciting the precepts. It requests that while taking this hand position a practitioner recites the precepts each morning and evening.

The aim of the system is then acknowledged:

> Improve your mind and body.

Mind and body are considered the two major areas that structure humankind and when integrated create a balanced life. These are the two diamonds that when brought together in balance, create the third diamond which is representative of the entire self or spirit. Practicing this system returns one to the true nature of the self – faultless, sparkling diamond.

With the names of the system and founder closing the creed:

Usui Reiki Ryôhô, the founder Usui Mikao.

Usui Reiki Ryôhô is the name of the method and literally translates as Usui Spiritual Healing Method. Usui Mikao is named as the founder of the system.

The five precepts are taught in the first level of the system of Reiki today and should be revisited constantly by the teacher and practitioner. The teachings are also universal, meaning that they are open to anyone regardless of their personal religious beliefs.

Source

The word 'precept' generally means 'rule of conduct' and there are many of these in Buddhism, some for monks and nuns and others for lay people. In Japanese Buddhism, there are five precepts or *gokai*. They exhort a Buddhist practitioner not to: kill, steal, commit adultery, tell lies, and not to drink intoxicants. These precepts, however, must not be confused with the system of Reiki's *gokai* even though some of the sentiments are similar.

Usui, as he was want to do, took a component of a well-established form and created his own non-religious version. It is more likely that the precepts are the layperson's version of the eight-fold path from Buddhism. The eight-fold path states that a practitioner must hold: right views, right thinking, right speech, right action, right way of life, right endeavor, right mindfulness and right meditation. The word 'right' according to Buddhist interpretation has specific connotations for a practitioner. Once a practitioner follows either the eight-fold path or the Reiki precepts the same quality of life can be experienced.

The first precepts taught by Usui were translated into his own words from an older set of Buddhist precepts. These precepts were initially from the early 9th century and were used daily in the practice of Shugendô – according to Suzuki san. They were a part of his first teachings that were then adjusted to become the five precepts – as we know them today. Usui is believed to have taught precepts from as early as 1915.

Within the context of Buddhism, at this time it was common for students to sit and write word for word their teacher's commentaries and contemplations. This appears to have also been the case with the precepts.[3] It is generally believed that the act of writing is yet another method to help internalize the text's meanings.

Apart from precepts there were also *gyosei, waka* (short poems) written by the Shinto Meiji Emperor (1852–1912), which were taught and practiced in similar ways to Usui's precepts. It is thought that their inclusion may well have been relevant to the times that Usui lived in. Today they are not widely studied – if at all. During the Meiji Emperor's reign, as well as using the Buddhist influenced Reiki precepts, the Shinto influenced *waka* would have been politically correct to use.

Rewards

These precepts appear to be practical reminders on how to get the most out of life by affirming correct attitudes but their secret is that they can affect humans in other, deeper ways.

It is the first line 'For today only' that establishes immediacy to the precepts, taking them further than being just five separate codes. Though they are called the five precepts, there are in fact six precepts; that first line 'For today only' is perhaps the most important of all codes to live by.

If seriously worked with, the precepts no longer become targets to be reached but are absorbed into the action of each moment, becoming an unconscious law. Their influence on one's thoughts becomes automatic. Eventually all that one does incorporates the principle 'For today only' and the five individual precepts. Therefore the benefits of practicing *gokai*, though deceptively simple, resound through all aspects of a practitioner's life.

Application

To apply the precepts on a daily basis make
sure you have your own copy. Write them
down from this book and place them where you
meditate or are likely to be reminded of them. The act
of writing can also be a useful process for the reason mentioned earlier. If you like, create multiple copies and place them around your
house and work environment to bring your focus back to them on a
regular basis.

Each of the precepts can be used in recitation, meditation and
contemplation. Below are some methods you may like to use to work
with the precepts to achieve a deeper interaction and connection
with them.

In *The Japanese Art of Reiki* a traditional version of a technique (*Hatsurei Hô*) that incorporates *waka* has been described under Chapter 6
Kokyû Hô – Breathing Techniques.[4] If you wish to experiment with
using *waka* it is also possible to replace the *gokai* with them in the
following methods.

Gokai Recitation

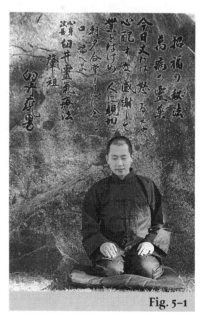

The recommendation
from the Reiki precepts is
that you must keep them
in mind and recite them
each morning and evening.
Recitation is a mental
process and learning a piece
by rote is useful but misses
an important element.
Either seated or standing,
try to *feel* each precept.
Allow the feeling of the
precept to soak through
you, working on a deeper
plane (Fig. 5–1). Traditionally,
in the *Usui Reiki Ryôhô*

Fig. 5–1

Gakkai, the *gokai* were recited three times at one sitting – this was called *gokai sansho.*

Gokai recitation aloud sounds powerful and coupled with feeling is a mighty tool to create inner change. Do not be alarmed if after time the sound lessens and turns inward, with recitation taking place in silence. Though it may not vocally sound as effective, you will sense that this change to inner practice is a natural development. Resonation with the precept itself will occur.

One recitation practice that is used in traditional Japanese forms and is listed in the *Usui Reiki Ryôhô Gakkai's* booklet, *shiori,* is *Nentatsu Hô.* This translates as 'a method for sending thoughts' and is a more formalized practice than the previous method. It is an ideal practice to use with *gokai* and is often taught in the first level of the system of Reiki to help rid one of bad habits or unwanted, yet ingrained, thought forms.

Sit in *seiza,* direct your gaze at the floor and bring your hands up to *gasshô,* breathing in a relaxed manner. Place one hand on your forehead and the other on the bump at the back of the head, the

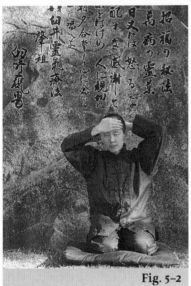

Fig. 5–2

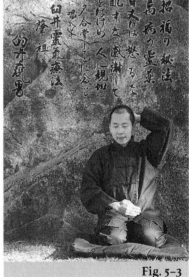

Fig. 5–3

medulla oblongata (Fig. 5–2). Recite one or all of the precepts for as long as five minutes. You may speak them out loud or repeat them to yourself. Afterwards remove your hand from the forehead and place it onto your *hara* (Fig. 5–3). Keep your other hand in place at the back of the head. Relax in this position, breathing regularly and end the practice with *gasshô*.

Gokai Meditation

Traditional practitioners of the system of Reiki including Usui's early teachings meditated on the precepts. Meditating on precepts is common to many traditions worldwide. Here is an example of how to meditate using *gokai*.

Before beginning, choose one of the precepts that you wish to work with. Sit in *seiza*, relax and focus your eyes toward the ground. *Gasshô*, then place your hands on your knees, palm face down. Bring your attention back from the daily occurrences and the rest of the room, letting your thoughts settle on the 'inner you' rather than the 'outer you' and the experiences attached

to that. Once you are sitting calmly allow your chosen precept to arise from within you. Let your own thoughts and experiences around this precept well up. Now bring the thoughts that you are experiencing into a positive relationship with the precept. Hold this sense of connection and inner understanding for as long as you need to absorb its significance (Fig. 5–4). *Gasshô* to finish.

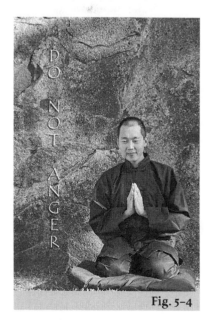

Fig. 5–4

Gokai Contemplation

To contemplate is a less formalized form of meditation that can be viewed as an excellent integrative tool between 'real life' and formal meditation. Life should not be separate from these precepts – the two must become one and contemplation aims at supporting practitioners in this aim.

People will find themselves contemplating various issues throughout their day while: waiting for the bus, sitting quietly in the evening, or slowly waking up. To contemplate, simply focus the mind on a thought and see what develops (Fig. 5–5).

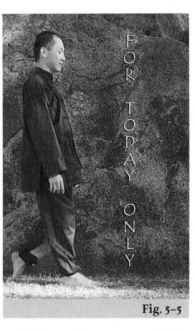

In the following precept table (Fig. 5–6) the precepts are listed on the left with inspirational thoughts about the precepts on the right. Choose a thought and see where it takes you. Find different levels of depth

Fig. 5–5

within the words. In your contemplation practice you may wish to create your own thoughts to focus on for each precept.

Questions

1. Do you currently live your life consciously? What are the advantages of bringing more consciousness into your daily life?
2. Have you ever replaced conscious living with other activities that were unsupportive of making yourself whole?
3. What 'rules' or precepts currently govern the actions that you undertake in your daily life? Take into consideration

Precept	Thought
For today only	*Ichi-go, ichi-e*: one encounter, one opportunity I am Tomorrow never arrives The past is behind me Now
Do not anger	*Wa*: harmony Anger is an out of control emotion I choose anger Anger doesn't express my true thoughts Anger is often confused with expressing myself An opposite of anger is balance
Do not worry	To worry is a reflection of my desire for attention. Worry is often confused with expressing concern Worry is a useless emotion that wastes inner Ki and therefore encourages ill health Worry is a repeated pattern learnt from my parents Worry is the inability to quieten my mind and experience peace An opposite of worry is faith Worry focuses on the past and future, in the Now there is no time for worry
Be humble	Thank you Accept both 'good' and 'bad' and move on I am my inner truth Humbleness cannot be claimed Know nothing
Be honest in your work	Daily practice My life is my work Perseverance Am I honest?
Be compassionate to yourself and others	*Uchu-rei*: Universal Mind Oneness Love Forgiveness Acceptance See life through the eyes of others Reach in and reach out

Fig. 5-6   The Five Precepts

your interaction with your parents, your colleagues, your friends, your partner, your children, your community and yourself.

4. Are these 'rules' relevant to, or supportive of, your lifestyle today?

5. Which of the Reiki precepts do you think is most significant to you at this point in your life? Why?

6 Kokyû Hô

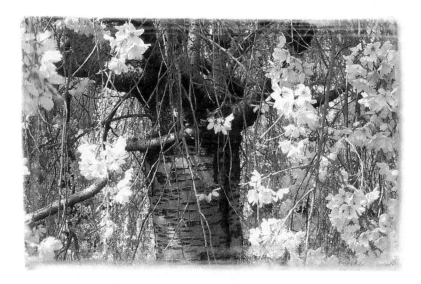

Kokyû Hô – breathing method

Description

Various techniques, including physical and
meditative practices, are taught throughout
the three levels of the system of Reiki. This chapter
focuses on the traditional self-healing *kokyû hô* techniques that stem from the system's beginnings in the first half of the
20th century.

    Kokyû hô, or breathing techniques, in the system of Reiki use breath coupled to both physical and energetic movement. Propelled along by Ki, the breath purposefully moves through the body. Breath is the essence of our earthly existence, without the function of breathing in and out we would die and our human experience would be over. It is no wonder that fundamental Reiki techniques, aiming to enrich existence by creating balance and wholeness, work with breath.

According to William Reed, author of *Ki*, Japanese use the word *naga-iki* to mean both 'long breath' and 'long life'. The concept is that each human is born with a pre-ordained number of breaths. When anger, distress, or fear are felt, breathing quickens – accordingly shortening life. When Ki flows freely in the body, breath is drawn and expelled with ease. The study of breathing in a relaxed and calm manner is therefore considered integral to a long and happy life. Sense this for yourself; stop reading and slowly breathe in and out. As the breath travels in and out of your body does it shudder and jump or is it one smooth movement? The more you practice *kokyû* techniques the freer that the breath moves thus extending your physical and mental wellness.

Four techniques will be described in full in this chapter. Rather than bombarding the reader with a great variety of techniques from different backgrounds,[5] essential techniques for self-practice – to clear and build a practitioner's energy – have been chosen.

There are three major techniques taught in the first level of the system that lie at its foundation. The first of these is a cleansing technique called *Kenyoku Hô*. Following that is *Jôshin Kokyû Hô*: a meditation to focus the mind using breath and; finally, *Seishin Toitsu*: a unifying the mind meditation. These are taught in traditional forms of the system of Reiki.

The last is a meditation taught in the second level of the system called *Hatsurei Hô*. In modern times it is practiced simply as a combination of the three aforementioned techniques. Instead, an original version of *Hatsurei Hô*, written by a student of Usui called Tomita Kaiji in 1933, has been included here.

Source

Kokyû techniques in Japan have been practiced namely in both religious and martial arts

practices with Usui being a serious practitioner of both traditions. Martial arts practices such as *Daito Ryu Jujitsu* and *aikidô* advocate that practices based on *kokyû* bring about an awareness of the whole. Such awareness is the result of a unified mind and body developed through *kokyû*.

After Usui's death in 1926, a number of techniques were taught under the auspices of the system of Reiki. Some of these techniques made their way to America in the late 1930s while others did not.

Rewards

The Japanese techniques are based on building the flow of Ki through the body's energetic pathways and strengthening the *hara* center using Reiki. This, in turn, energetically clears the body, mind and heart thus raising a practitioner's vibration level enabling one to become lighter and lighter.

To become one with this energetic flow one must learn to let go – something that humans struggle constantly against. Surrendering to this flow can result in clarity of thought, renewed physical strength, calmness, reduced stress levels, a sense of connectedness as well as the easing of conditions such as insomnia, depression and addiction. A practitioner may also experience physical healing with acute and even chronic illness. The immune system strengthens allowing the body to fight off illness easier and an accelerated speed of healing is often observed – making the practice an excellent form of first aid treatment.

> Ki breathing improves delivery of oxygen and nutrients and accelerates the removal of toxins from bodily tissues. Both the liver and the kidneys become stronger and more efficient resulting in improved health and resistance to disease.[6]

To consciously let go will also change your perceptions about how you live your life. This is partly due to the realization when practicing *kokyû* techniques that the source of life is unlimited. Holding on to people, possessions and thoughts will only imprison you. Learning to let go of expectation, drama and the need for total control will allow you to run back into the flow of the universal river of life. In your practice attempt to return to the essence of letting go rather than trying to take on new philosophies or fashions.

Something that is always important to remember is; how you approach your meditation determines what you get out of it. Your level of dedication will deliver your appropriate rewards. If your preparation is focused and clear and the method exact, then the aim can be achieved within time. It comes from your work – not from a magical potion that is handed to you. This self-responsibility is at the core of the system of Reiki and is an empowering force that will teach you what true magic is.

Application

Kenyoku Hô

Kenyoku – dry bath
Hô – method

Before beginning any energetic practice a practitioner needs to be in a correct frame of mind and state of body. To achieve this, the technique *Kenyoku Hô* is performed. *Kenyoku Hô* is a form of cleansing called *misogi*: a common Shinto practice that can take many forms including standing under rushing waterfalls.

Shintoism is particularly concerned with purity – at Shinto shrines for example there is always a place for hand and mouth washing. The basic teachings of Shintoism believe that humans are originally pure and that there is in essence nothing that divides humans from *kami* (gods). *Kami*, though, do not like dirtiness and humans suffer the constant challenge of cleaning away the soil that sticks to one's body and mind to return to the state of cleanliness or, if you like, godliness.

Kenyoku Hô is in many ways a symbolic practice as much as an energetic one. It is called dry bathing as it physically imitates some of the actions of cleansing the body while bathing. The physical action in conjunction with the breath stimulates the clearing of energy along the arms and through the major organs. Clearing the arms supports a practitioner in channeling more Ki through them, which is very beneficial for palm-healing. The organs form the body's engine and cleansing them is a tuning up that should be a regular occurrence. Symbolically, it brushes away dirt accumulated by the mind eventuating in a practitioner feeling light, fresh and renewed before beginning a practice. This energetic form of cleansing can be thought of as a practitioner's first step to healing.

> *Kenyoku Hô* can be practiced on its own or as a precursor to another energetic practice.
>
> To begin, follow through with the six principles to ready yourself for practice: decide upon the technique/s, sit or stand (depending on the chosen follow up technique), fix your eyes on the floor, release all tension from the body, bring the mental focus to the *hara*, and allow the hands to rise in *gasshô*. There are two parts to this technique.
>
> Place your right hand on the left shoulder (where the collarbone and shoulder meet) (Fig. 6–1). Breathe in and on the out breath sweep your right hand diagonally down and across the torso to the right hip and off the body (Fig. 6–2). In this large sweep the energy from the left shoulder, heart, stomach and liver is cleared.

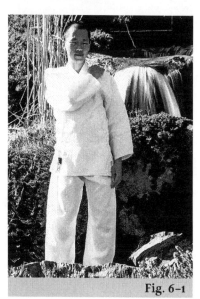

Fig. 6–1

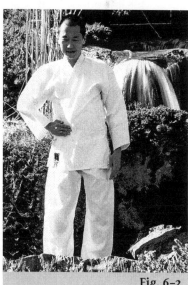

Fig. 6–2

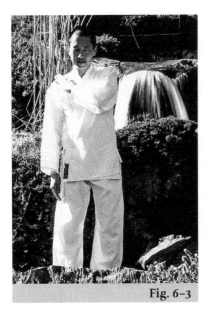

Fig. 6-3

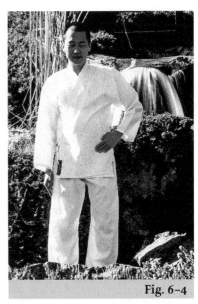

Fig. 6-4

Breathe in again, this time placing your left hand onto the right shoulder (Fig. 6–3). Breathe out and at the same time sweep diagonally down and across the body to the left hip and off the body (Fig. 6–4). Now the energy from the left shoulder, heart, stomach and spleen has been cleared.

To finish the first half of this technique, place the right hand on the left shoulder once again (Fig. 6–5) sweeping down to the right hip (Fig. 6–6).

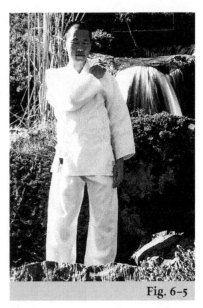

Fig. 6-5

The second half of the technique begins by placing your bent left elbow against your side with your forearm held straight out in front, horizontal to the ground. Your left palm is flat,

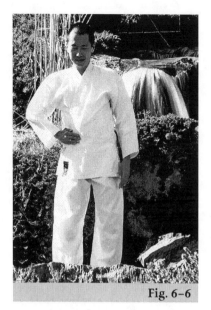

Fig. 6–6

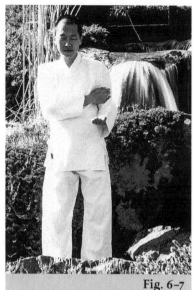

Fig. 6–7

facing upward and level to the ground as if you are balancing a plate on it. Place your right hand at top of the left arm (Fig. 6–7). Breathe in and on the out breath – sweep downward along the arm through the crook of the elbow, across the palm to the fingertips and off the hands (Fig. 6–8).

Repeat this action with the other side of the body. Your bent right elbow is against your side and your forearm is straight out in front, horizontal to the ground. Your

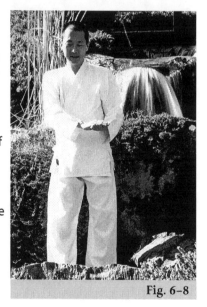

Fig. 6–8

right palm is also flat. Place your left hand at the top of the right arm (Fig. 6–9). Breathe in and on the out breath sweep downward along the arm to the fingertips and off the hands (Fig. 6–10).

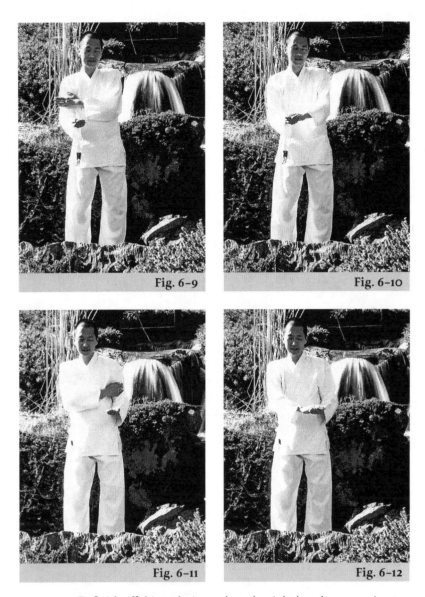

Fig. 6–9

Fig. 6–10

Fig. 6–11

Fig. 6–12

To finish off this technique place the right hand once again at the top of the left arm (Fig. 6–11) and brush down along the left arm to the fingertips and off the hands (Fig. 6–12).

Once finished, bring your hands up in *gasshô* to round off the technique.

Jôshin Kokyû Hô

Jôshin – focusing the mind
Kokyû – breath, respiration
Hô – method

Meditations may work with any number of focal points including the breath, mantras, physical or energetic points, and visual images. All are, in fact, single pointed meditation practices where a practitioner focuses on one point to enter a specified meditative state.

Jôshin Kokyû Hô is a single pointed meditation focusing on using Ki driven breath to sense, and develop the *hara*. There may be many responses to these meditations: sometimes physical, energetic or emotional. These sensations, surprisingly, are not the aim of the meditation but the side effects of the practice. This meditation should be taken further than these responses as it is there that true understanding takes place. This can only occur after much practice.

To reach your inner core through meditation, you must first learn the practicalities of the meditation itself and then create a regular, daily routine. Though you may think, 'I am now going to meditate deeper than a monk' when you seat yourself – it is generally not possible. Each practice has an 'aim' and then within that aim are the machinations of practice itself. Different levels of meditation exist and to immediately submerge into the deepest level takes great stamina and determination, over many years.

It is wise to remember this, as it is a deceivingly simple process to 'try' meditations. What exactly are you achieving with this? Go further than trying something out – practice and experience it, take it beyond words. It is suggested that *Jôshin Kokyû Hô* be practiced from six months up to one year before moving on to the following meditation in *The Japanese Art of Reiki: Seishin Toitsu*.

Before beginning the meditation practice it is useful to observe the cleansing routine of *Kenyoku Hô*. Prior to this remember to always practice the six principles for preparation: know your technique, sit in *seiza* with your eyes gazing at the floor, release all tension from the body, bring the mental focus to the *hara*, and allow the hands to rise in *gasshô*.

Once you are ready place your hands on your knees, with the

palms facing upwards (Fig. 6–13). Begin by breathing in through the nose (Fig. 6–14). With this breath travels the power of Ki. Bring the breath down through the body to the *hara* and fill it with

energy. On the out breath expand the energy out through the body, then via your skin and expanding the energy out into your surroundings (Fig. 6–15). It is like blowing up a balloon. You are taking in the energy on the in breath and then on the out breath you're filling out the balloon: your body and the space it inhabits.

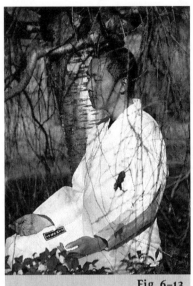

Fig. 6–13

Continue breathing in through the nose, down to the *hara* and expanding the Ki out through the

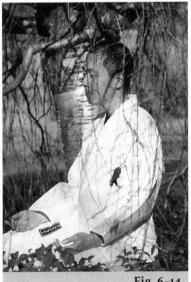

Fig. 6–14

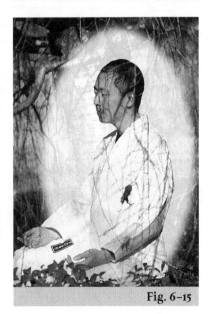

Fig. 6–15

body on the out breath for anywhere from five minutes up to an hour. If you begin to feel dizzy then finish the technique. This is the body adjusting to your new practice and can possibly be caused by energy being cleared. Over the following weeks slowly build up your amount of practice time.

When you are finished bring the hands up into *gasshô*.

Seishin Toitsu

Seishin – spirit, mind, soul, intention
Toitsu – to unite, unify (to make one)

The *Seishin Toitsu* meditation takes the breath through a specific pattern in the body. By physically bringing together the left and right, the meditation aims at creating a unified self. Being a single-pointed meditation one major benefit is the clearing of the mind. Due to its focus on the hands it develops their sensitivity creating excellent palm-healing antenna, and its focus on the *hara* once again builds and strengthens the Earth Ki connection.

Before beginning the meditation practice it is useful to observe the cleansing routine of *Kenyoku Hô*. Prior to this remember to always practice the six principles for preparation: know your technique, sit in *seiza* with your eyes gazing at the floor, release all tension from the body, bring the mental focus to the *hara*, and allow the hands to rise in *gasshô*.

With the hands still in *gasshô* (Fig. 6–16), focus your mind on the *hara*. On the in breath begin to bring the energy into your hands and feel it moving along your arms, down though your body and into the *hara*. On the out breath visualize energy moving from the *hara*

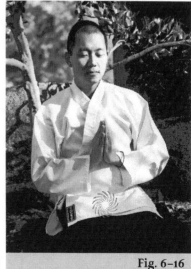

Fig. 6–16

back up through the body and then out through the arms and finally the hands (Fig. 6–17).

Continue breathing in and out, moving the Ki from your hands through the torso down to the *hara* and back again. Initially it can be difficult to feel the Ki traveling along this pathway; you may feel your Ki moves slowly, irregularly or that your breath is not long enough. To simplify the action – place your intent at your hands as you breathe in and then

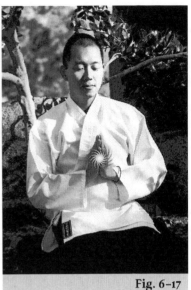

Fig. 6-17

immediately focus on the *hara*. Do not take the Ki on a journey through the arms and torso – just know that it is at the *hara*. Repeat this with the out breath. Place your intent at the *hara* and then focus on the hands knowing that the Ki has moved to that point on the out breath.

This practice can take anywhere from five minutes up to an hour. In the same manner as the previous technique, build on the time in which this technique is practiced.

Once a practitioner feels confident with the former technique of *Jôshin Kokyû Hô*, progression can be made to *Seishin Toitsu*. *Jôshin Kokyû Hô* is practiced in preparation for the following practice of *Seishin Toitsu*. Therefore the effectiveness of *Seishin Toitsu* will depend upon the strength of the foundation created by practicing *Jôshin Kokyû Hô*.

The joining of these two techniques (with *Kenyoku Hô* always preceding the routine) is a complete technique taught in the second level of the system: in its modern form it is called *Hatsurei Hô*. To help you tap into the more traditional self-practice methods an older version of *Hatsurei Hô* has been included below.

Hatsurei Hô

Hatsu – to generate
Rei – spirit
Hô – method

The concept of *Hatsurei Hô* is to generate greater amounts of Ki in the body. In 1933, a student of Usui called Tomita Kaiji wrote a book describing techniques that he taught to his students. His major technique was *Hatsurei Hô*. It is not specifically a breathing technique like its modern relative (though naturally one does breathe throughout the technique) but rather a single pointed meditation using words.

Tomita uses *gyosei*, a form of poetry (called *waka*) written by the Meiji Emperor, as the meditation's focus point. The Meiji Emperor is known to have written around 100,000 *waka* during his lifetime – many of them of a spiritual nature. Poetry has been a common and natural part of Japanese life in the past. To be able to write and recite poetry was considered the sign of a cultured education.

First sit in *seiza* with your eyes lowered to the floor, feeling relaxed and calm. The technique then begins with a variation on the modern *Seishin Toitsu*. Bring the hands into *gasshô* (Fig. 6–18) with the objective of gathering Ki from the heart and bringing it into the palms of the hands. Hold the hands together lightly without using force from the arms or shoulders. Continue to focus on bringing Ki from the heart into the hands (Fig. 6–19). Though the original technique does not mention it, this Ki movement naturally occurs in conjunction with the movement of breath.

The next step is to unify and purify the mind with the recitation of *waka*.

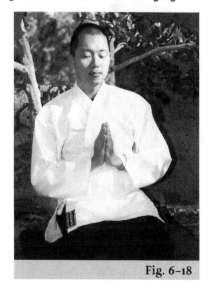

Fig. 6–18

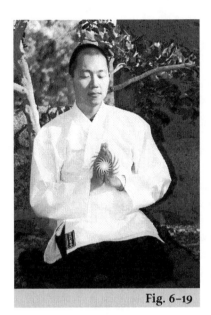

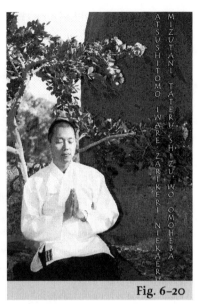

Fig. 6–19

Fig. 6–20

The purpose is to feel at one with the true essence of the *waka* (Fig. 6–20).

Here is one example of the Meiji Emperor's *waka* that was used by Mikao Usui[7]:

> Thinking of lowly people standing in a boiling hot paddy field
> I hesitate to utter 'It's hot.'

Here is the Japanese pronunciation of this particular *waka*. You may like to experience reciting it in Japanese:

> *Atsushitomo iware zarikeri niekaeru*
> *Mizutani tateru shizu wo omoheba*

Japanese Reiki teacher Mochizuki Toshitaka, who was responsible for reprinting Tomita's 1933 book in 1999, notes next to the technique *Hatsurei Hô* that modern practitioners should feel free to choose sayings, sentences or visualizations that are more appropriate to their times. One other poem that might be interesting for recitation is the one from the notebook of Mikao

Usui that is said to be an extract from an eighth century Buddhist prayer on the nature of impermanence[8].

> *Like stars, mists and candle flames*
> *Mirages, dewdrops and water bubbles*
> *Like dreams, lightning and clouds.*
> *In that way I will view all existence.*

Tomita goes on to write that if you follow the previous steps and stay focused on the palms of your hands they will start to become warm. He describes their tingling sensation as comparable to an electrical current. Even if the sensations are weak at first, he states that they will become stronger as you keep concentrating. This technique should be practiced for at least thirty minutes, building gradually to one hour.

Questions

1. Do you feel limited in any areas of your life? Which areas? How does that make you feel?
2. Do you realize that with each in breath you are drawing an unlimited supply of energy into your body? To experience abundance consciously, focus on your breath.
3. What sensations do you experience, physically and/or emotionally, as you sense the breath move into the body and then out again? Write them down. Continue to do this at intervals during your practice and then compare them after six months of *kokyû hô* practice.
4. Do you consider yourself a radiant being? This is your true nature waiting to be discovered.
5. How long can you see yourself sitting in meditation each day? Visualize yourself successfully meditating.

7 Tenohira

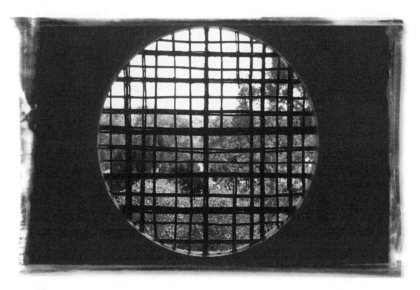

Tenohira – palm-healing

Description

Tenohira is the act of supporting Ki to emanate
from the palms of the hands for healing purposes.

Placing the hands on the body as self-treatment is yet
another aspect to healing the self within the system of Reiki. The
practitioner places hands on or just off the body with the intent that
Ki passes from them to the intended body part. The Ki is not pushed
or forced from the hands, it is actually drawn through them by the

receiving body. Once the body senses the Ki, it takes it where it needs and wants it. So, although the hands may be placed on what is considered an area of need there are more elements at play deciding on its direction and use.

The reason for placing the hands on or near the body is to allow Ki to clear stagnant energy, ultimately resulting in free flowing Ki. The added physicality of *tenohira* has its own unique rewards for the practitioner. A person who practices Reiki is not a Reiki 'healer' but a 'practitioner' for the simple reason that it is not the practitioner that is 'doing' the healing rather the universal Ki attempting to flow as freely as possible.

Hand positions generally cover the head, torso and limbs. It is beneficial for a practitioner to initially learn specific hand positions so that there is a sound basis to deviate from, once confidence and energetic knowledge is gained.

Tenohira is taught in the first level of the system of Reiki.

Source

Palm-healing has a global history that extends throughout the ages. Religious groups and even monarchies (using their 'Royal Touch') have often claimed exclusive rights to these gifts, yet the truth is that each person has his or her own innate ability to heal. This is how the human body has evolved. For example, once cut, the skin develops a protective layer – the scab. This scab offers protection while skin reconstruction is diligently taking place underneath. Eventually the scab peels away exposing a perfectly new and ready-to-wear skin. Fever is another amazing gift the human body has developed over time. Firstly, it warns that inflammation is present. Secondly, it creates the antidote by kicking the immune system into action. Even emotionally the body moves into damage control by finding all manner of ways to continue to function effectively under extreme situations. An example of this is the fight or flight response that humans are hard wired with. Under stress the hypothalamus is stimulated, thus releasing chemicals to prepare the body to either run away or stay and fight. These are the natural abilities of excellently programmed bodies.

Touch is another naturally accessible component of a body's holistic medicine chest. With touch you allow energy to be drawn and transferred via your palms. If you stub your toe your first instinct is to hold it … and then scream.

Historically, Usui taught *tenohira*. The spiritual teachings, including meditations, appear to have been his earliest teachings with palm-healing being added on in his later years. Once Usui began working with lay students he taught in a more formalized manner. Approached by Japanese naval officers, he began instructing the use of *tenohira* as a form of 'first aid'. Palm-healing initially consisted of using five head positions and then the practitioner would intuitively place hands elsewhere on the body. Therefore, *tenohira* was taught to students to help themselves and others. The knowledge of where to place the hands on the body was formalized by Usui's student, a naval surgeon, Hayashi Chûjirô. Hayashi went on to begin a formal treatment centre where clients could visit for healing. His practitioners worked in pairs on clients with one treating the head and the other the *hara*: balancing the mind and body at once.

The great popularity of palm-healing in Japan in the early 1900s meant that it was being experimented with across the board. A friend and student of Usui called Eguchi Toshihiro was involved with different groups working with *tenohira*. As principal of a school in Nagano he invited Nishida Tenko (Fig. 7-1) to give a presentation. Nishida founded a community called *Ittôen* in 1904. This community still exists today and is comprised of those wishing to seek a life of no possessions, serving in a spirit of penitence. They believe that when human beings live in accordance with the way of nature, they are accepted and enabled to live, even without owning things and even without

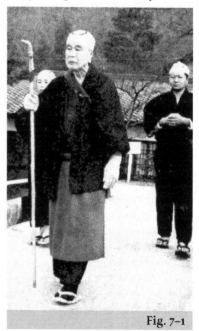

Fig. 7-1

converting labor into money. Today the *Ittôen* community consists of around one hundred members with their leader being Nishida's grandson, Takeshi. The *Ittôen* members traditionally practiced a form of palm-healing acquired directly from Eguchi who visited the community several times. Today some families still practice palm-healing but there is no official practice within the community. Miss Endo, (aged around ninety-seven in 1994) an original *Ittôen* student of Eguchi ca 1929 or 1930, previously made her 'evening rounds' with palm-healing in the community before her passing.

Many of Eguchi's hand positions are listed in his book *Tenohira Ryôji Nyûmon* (*Introduction to Healing with the Palms*) written in 1930. These positions are similar in nature to those listed in the manuals of the *Usui Reiki Ryôhô Gakkai* and Hayashi Chûjirô.

Tomita Kaiji, another student of Usui, also describes many hand positions from his own system in his book from 1933.

Today, palm-healing has been popularized around the world due largely to the system of Reiki. With this increasing recognition, awareness about the body's natural abilities grows with each day.

Rewards

Treating the self is fundamental to healing on a global level. If each person tapped into their human potential and allowed transformation to occur there would be no need for cures, and death would be a natural phenomenon experienced from the wisdom of wholeness.

Connection occurs within the universe in many ways – one of these is touch. Touch is the energetic union created by placing hands on or near the body. When applying the system of Reiki the effect of touch is amplified. The clear intent of a Reiki practitioner ensures that greater amounts of spiritual energy are activated in and around the body. Once awareness is placed on the healing ability of one's own body that ability is strengthened.

The actual placing of the hands on or near the body is a ritual. This 'hands-on' rite is the permission that a practitioner gives one's self to allow healing to occur: it triggers the release of resistance. The responsibility of a practitioner is to let go and allow the Ki to move and not to try to control the process – this would only limit it. Your body's focus is on survival and it will want to deal firstly with issues that compromise its survival. For example, you may believe you need to work on your ability to communicate with others but your body draws the majority of the energy to your left knee. You are not aware of any problem you have with your knee but you must accept that your body knows best. You do not consciously decide upon these things. This lesson is a superb way for you to begin to understand, and to begin to incorporate into your life, the concept of letting go: succumbing to your inner knowledge and knowing that what is best for you will occur. Now take this journey just one step further – allow it to happen.

A practitioner is solely a channel for Ki, consequently his or her energy is not being 'given'. If this were the case then practitioners might feel that their own Ki should become depleted. A practitioner's own energy levels are in fact enhanced and rebalanced by simply allowing Ki to be activated in the body and drawn through the palms. This concept of Ki work being out of a practitioner's direct control also assures a certain level of safety, as universal energy is incapable of making mistakes.

When energy moves there is the possibility that you are going to undergo change. Some adjustments may be pleasant while others may be difficult to move through. It may even be necessary for you to endure the re-emergence of scars of the body, mind or spirit. This is a wonderful thing and is called a clearing: energy attempting to move and/or dissolve stagnant energy. You may feel the energy actually moving as you place your hands on specific positions. Once you can sense energy in motion, remain there until the Ki movement wanes. This energy is doing what the body needs.

The time you spend each day placing hands on your body is a loving experience that is totally about you. Self-nurturing contains true healing – it creates a sense of wholeness that may not often be experienced. Many people have little time to care for themselves, being so involved with the outer world. To take time out for yourself – acknowledging that you are important – is totally healing and supportive.

The sense of touch and immediacy of Ki sensation was understood by the Japanese in the 1920s to be of immense value. It is something that a person can know and initiate for their benefit and for the benefit of others. Touching is commonly used in Reiki because physical touch (without sexual intimacy) is unusual in most modern societies. To be touched without any other motivation than love is a wonderful healing process in itself.

In the West there has been a great importance attached to *tenohira* in the system of Reiki. This has mostly been focused on helping others rather than the self. *Tenohira* on the self is a totally natural way to experience life and the system reminds people of this generous innate ability. Suzuki san's aide states, 'Healing becomes not something you do or give – but what you are.'

Application

It is possible to use *tenohira* anytime and anyplace but the intention, and therefore the effect, is stronger when the basics are taken seriously. As with everything in life, the more we put into something the more we get out of it.

A treatment can include anything from placing hands on one area of the body in a 'first aid' type situation to a full treatment. In a complete treatment, the practitioner begins at the head and works down through the body covering as much of it as possible. For a short treatment or for 'first aid' it is possible to use Reiki on the train, at work, in the shower or …anywhere. Consequently *tenohira* can take anything from a couple of minutes in length to an hour or longer – though setting aside a specific amount of time in a daily routine will create the most effective self-treatment practice.

Tenohira can be practiced as often as you wish although it is recommended that a practitioner create a daily routine. Initially most students are given a specific time frame to work within. This is generally a twenty-one-day period that includes half an hour of *tenohira* practice on the self a day. For this you may wish to begin with the Full Body Treatment and once you are more experienced working with Ki you advance to the Head Treatment. At any time you may experiment with the technique *Gedoku Hô*.

The venue for working on yourself should preferably be quiet. For a complete treatment you can either be seated (in *seiza*) or lying down. It is possible to create a whole experience by lying on a yoga mat, futon, lounge or comfortable floor in an undisturbed area. Try not to practice in bed, as it is likely that you will fall asleep though you may close your eyes if you prefer. During a long treatment the body can cool down when working with Reiki so it is wise to either place a blanket over yourself or keep one handy. If you wish, play tranquil music, light candles and enjoy soft lighting – why not? You are about to be kind to yourself.

Do not press too hard when placing hands on the body as it is the not the pressure that affects healing but the movement of Ki. For this reason the hands may also be held off the body. When holding hands off the body intuitively sense the connection between your hands and your body – once you have found the strongest energetic bond hold your hands at that location. As you spend more time working on the self an inner guidance moves your hands to the appropriate positions and placements. There is no rationale behind this. Obviously an element of common sense can guide you too – never place your hands directly on burns or extremely painful spots. If you were practicing on a client your hands would naturally be placed off the body on private or sensitive parts; yet, on the self this is not necessary. In fact, touching your own culturally taboo body parts can be healing in itself. There are no physical parts that do not love touch. The decision to place hands on or off the body has many variables and the ultimate decision can be made through experience only. Many people find that more can be sensed via the hands when they are held off the body. Though the actual physical sensation of touch is, in itself, a valuable healing tool.

The length of time spent at each position can be timed if necessary to begin with but it is better to immediately begin working at developing your senses. Though you may not instantaneously sense something, leave hands in that position for a couple of minutes. This will give you time to adapt to the position and to pick up Ki movement. Beginners generally need more time to adjust to each position. If hands are moved too quickly from position to new position little benefit may be received. If sensations are experienced, remain in that position for as long as they occur – this can be anywhere from a couple of minutes up to half an hour

The actual sensations felt from the practice are side effects

– granted they can be useful, offering encouragement and indicating where and when Ki is or is not flowing. They can indicate where to practice and when Ki sensations lessen but they cannot signify why this is so. Any judgment about one's health made due to these sensations would be misguided. That would indicate the human need to control the situation from a rational and, consequently, limited viewpoint. Humans are just one small part of the universe and instead of attempting to control its flow they need to let go and become a part of it. Ki heals as it flows and the greater the flow the more enhanced the healing – this is all that you need to remember. Exactly what it is healing is unimportant. This is a lesson in letting go and releases the need to satisfy a hungry ego.

Do be careful in the terminology you use for yourself. You are neither 'blocked' nor 'open' as these are judgmental statements that set you up to experience Ki in a certain way. To be totally 'blocked' would mean that you are surely dead and to be entirely 'open' would suggest that enlightenment has been and gone. It is unlikely that either of these statements is true if you are reading this book.

There are many metaphysical suggestions as to what these hand positions 'do'. These proposals are either culturally biased or are based on New Age terminology. Remember Ki moves wherever it wants rather than where you choose to believe it does. Metaphysical judgments in this case are there to flatter the ego rather than to aid healing. Many believe that the knowledge that these metaphysical concepts offer give the practitioner additional insight. This should perhaps be so but is problematic for two main reasons; the metaphysical concept is either extremely broad or generalized – not being a result of direct experience (but rather a book), or it is the experience of someone who has 'diagnosed' the situation (energy diagnosis is always subjective). Taking the human element out of healing with Ki will assure a smoother and less complex process that will ultimately be far more beneficial.

As with every practice mentioned in this book it is integral you have a clear understanding of what it is you are about to do. Be confident in your practice and you will be less distracted – resulting in a more successful practice. Focus, therefore, helps one to work effectively; yet, if a *tenohira* treatment on the self is a whole hour – how does this work? The mind is likely to drift away and begin to imagine the shopping list or where a lost sock might be. This does not mean that the palm-healing is not working. It does however mean that one is less focused, possibly resulting in lesser levels of Ki moving through the body. A good thing to remember is that Ki is perpetually in motion, even in what may seem a totally stagnant area. The slightest intent behind *tenohira* will be effective to some degree. The simple act of placing hands on or near the body gives that intent and consequently a trigger for Ki to move is set in action. *Tenohira* will always be working at something even if its results are not immediately felt.

Know that you may have some discomfort from the treatment later in the day or over the next couple of days. This is a good sign as it means that the Reiki is starting to move things in the body. If you feel like laughing or crying during *tenohira* then just let it out – this is a release and the form that it can take is unique to each person. If you experience reactions to your work make sure that you continue practicing *tenohira* to encourage the clearing. To help support the body's clearing process also drink lots of water: this will remove toxins and aid you in feeling grounded.

To relax into a treatment is very important. When you begin, breathe down into the *hara* at the abdomen. Do not force this, but breathe in a relaxed manner allowing the breath to enter and leave the body freely. The reason for this deep breathing is twofold. One: it gets the body to fill and release. This supports the physical body to unwind on the out breath. Two: it is also an action for the mind to follow. If you have something single-pointed to do, the mind naturally slows, eventually – allowing it to let go. It is not necessary to continue breathing in this fashion throughout the whole technique – it is simply a tool to aid the process of letting go. The more relaxed that you feel, the easier you will draw Ki through you.

Some important points to know when practicing *tenohira* on the self:

- *Tenohira* may be used as first aid and can therefore be practiced anywhere at anytime.
- Keep a daily practice routine and then add to it whenever *tenohira* is required in a specific situation.
- Hands may be placed on or just off the body.
- Be guided by your hands. Stay as long as your hands

indicate you to do so. Do be careful that you do not move too fast, consequently missing out on the sensation of Ki movement.

- Do not try to force the energy: learn to let go instead.
- Try not to diagnose your sensations. Know that some areas draw more Ki than others. There is neither a positive nor negative aspect to this.
- Do not judge your experience.
- Stay as focused as possible on what you are doing and know that Reiki will always be working on something.
- Discomfort or ill health can be the body clearing itself. Continue to practice *tenohira* to encourage this.
- Drink lots of water to support clearing.
- Relax and enjoy yourself.

Begin the routine with the six principles to ready yourself for practice: decide upon your practice, sit, softly gaze with the eyes at the floor, release all tension from the body, bring the mental focus to the *hara*, and allow the hands to rise in *gasshô*. You may now lie down and close the eyes if you wish.

Kenyoku Hô may be practiced as a cleansing practice before beginning any of these *tenohira* techniques.

Hand Poses

The hands are held slightly cupped and relaxed with *tenohira*. They mold to the body being both firm and flexible at the same time. Various positions in which to hold the hands can be used:

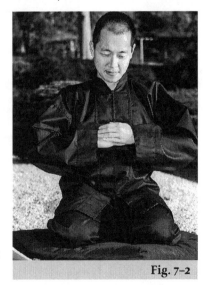

1. One hand on top of the other. They are placed either on the body or just off the body (Fig. 7–2).

Fig. 7–2

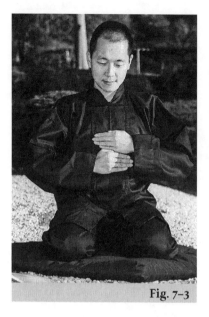

Fig. 7–3

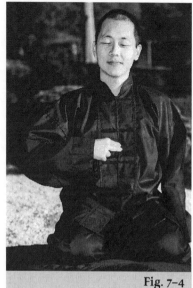

Fig. 7–4

2. Both hands placed next to each other. They are placed either on the body or just off the body (Fig. 7–3).

3. Focusing with the fingers of one hand on a specific area. This is generally performed directly on the body (Fig. 7–4).

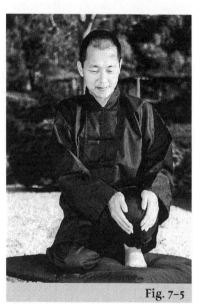

4. Enclose a particular body part or region with both hands. They are placed either on the body or just off the body (Fig. 7–5).

Fig. 7–5

5. Each hand placed on a separate part of the body. They are placed either on the body or just off the body. This pose is

generally used to create a sense of balance; for example, when the forehead and *hara* are held (a balancing of mind and body) (Fig. 7–6).

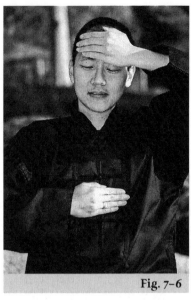

Fig. 7–6

Full Body Treatment

This procedure covers the entire body with hand placements and is an excellent beginner's guideline (Fig. 7–7 to Fig. 7–45). It is possible to use alternative positions such as those listed under Alternative Leg Positions (Fig. 7–46 to Fig. 7–50). Many beginners practice the Full Body Treatment first, later graduating to the Head Treatment on page 116: a more intuitive practice. In reality, no hand positions are ever totally set, as energy does not acknowledge human rules. A practitioner must learn to work intuitively and to do so a strong foundation, as is provided here, is integral. This entire treatment can be practiced from half an hour to as long as the practitioner deems necessary. The positions may be thought of as ir-

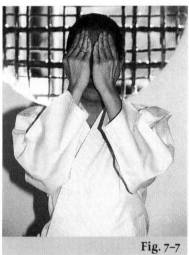

Fig. 7–7

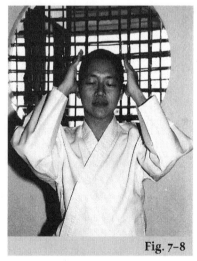

Fig. 7–8

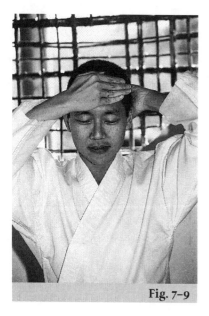

Fig. 7–9

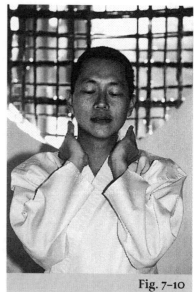

Fig. 7–10

relevant in the long run but are an integral first step along the road to personal discovery and better health. If you find that time is limited and you cannot fulfill the entire treatment you can skip the limbs.

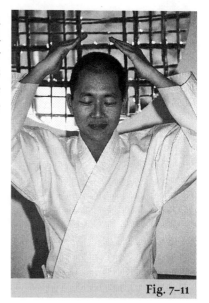

Head

1. The eyes and forehead (*zentô bu*) (Fig. 7–7)
2. Both temples (*sokutô bu*) (Fig. 7–8)
3. The back of the head (*medulla oblongata*) and forehead (*kôtô bu*) (Fig. 7–9)
4. Either side of the neck (*enzui bu*) (Fig. 7–10)
5. The crown (*tôchô bu*) (Fig. 7–11)

Fig. 7–11

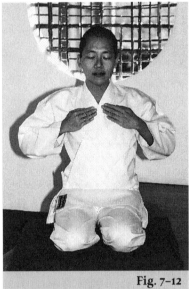

Fig. 7–12

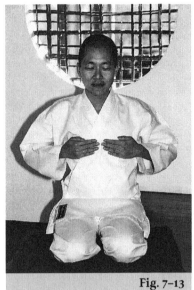

Fig. 7–13

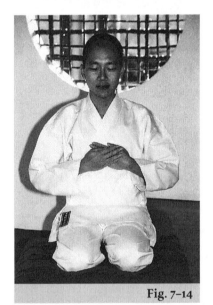

Fig. 7–14

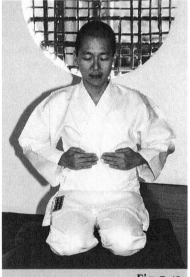

Fig. 7–15

Front Torso
6. Upper chest (Fig. 7–12)
7. Chest (Fig. 7–13)

8. Heart (Fig. 7–14)
9. Ribs/Lungs (Fig. 7–15)

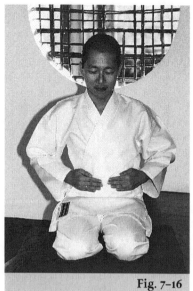

Fig. 7–16

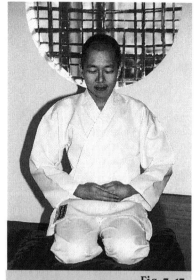

Fig. 7–17

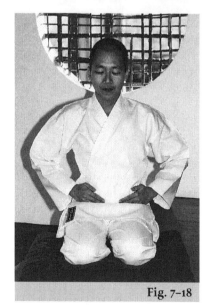

Fig. 7–18

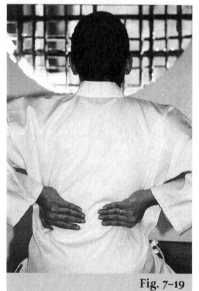

Fig. 7–19

10. Spleen/Liver (Fig. 7–16)
11. *Hara* (Fig. 7–17)
12. Ovaries/Testes (Fig. 7–18)

Back Torso
13. Back of ribs (Fig. 7–19)

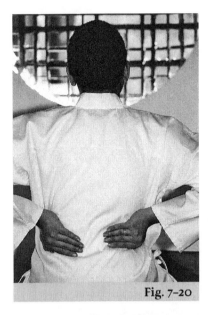

Fig. 7-20

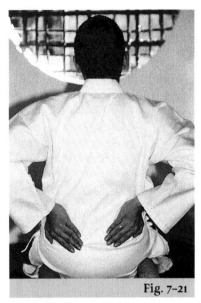

Fig. 7-21

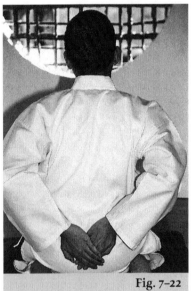

Fig. 7-22

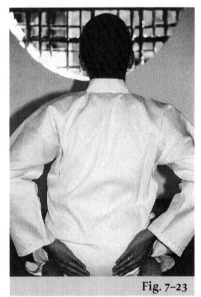

Fig. 7-23

14. Kidneys (Fig. 7–20)
15. Back of *hara* (Fig. 7–21)

16. Tailbone (Fig. 7–22)
17. Bottom (Fig. 7–23)

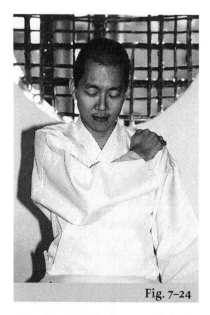

Fig. 7–24

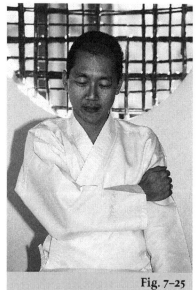

Fig. 7–25

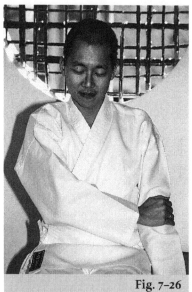

Fig. 7–26

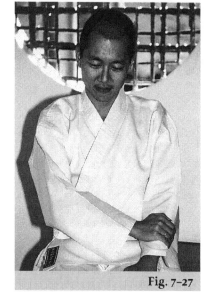

Fig. 7–27

Limbs – Left Arm
18. Left shoulder (Fig. 7–24)
19. Left bicep (Fig. 7–25)

20. Left elbow (Fig. 7–26)
21. Left forearm (Fig. 7–27)

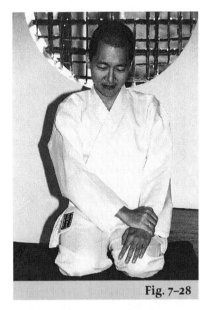

Fig. 7–28

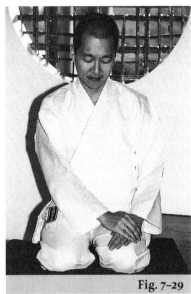

Fig. 7–29

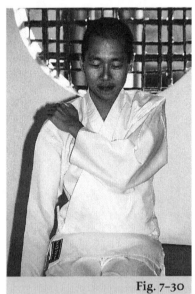

Fig. 7–30

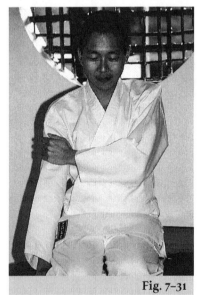

Fig. 7–31

22. Left wrist (Fig. 7–28)
23. Left hand (Fig. 7–29)

Right Arm
24. Right shoulder (Fig. 7–30)
25. Right bicep (Fig. 7–31)

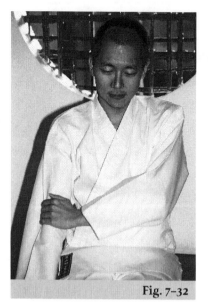

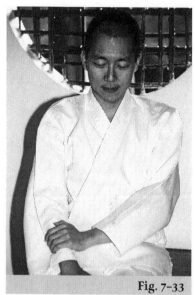

Fig. 7-32

Fig. 7-33

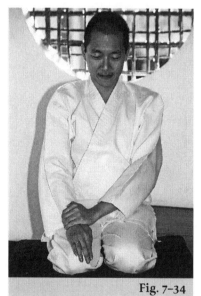

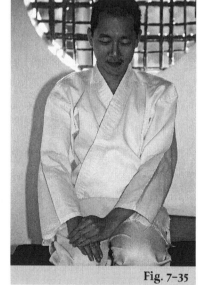

Fig. 7-34

Fig. 7-35

26. Right elbow (Fig. 7–32)
27. Right forearm (Fig. 7–33)

28. Right wrist (Fig. 7–34)
29. Right hand (Fig. 7–35)

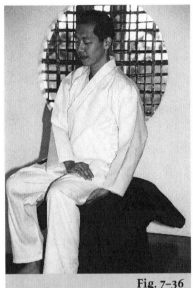

Fig. 7–36

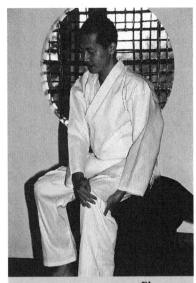

Fig. 7–37

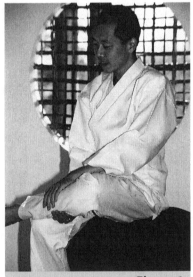

Fig. 7–38

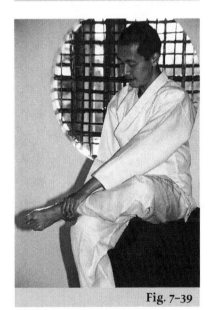

Fig. 7–39

Left leg
30. Left thigh (Fig. 7–36)
31. Left knee (Fig. 7–37)

32. Left shin (Fig. 7–38)
33. Left ankle (Fig. 7–39)
34. Left foot (Fig. 7–40)

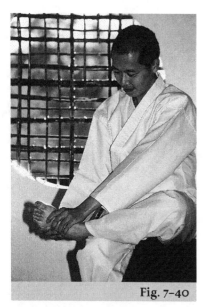

Fig. 7–40

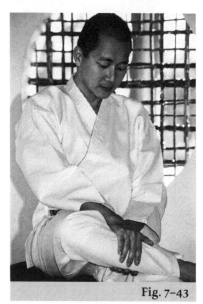

Fig. 7–41

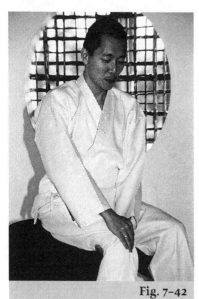

Fig. 7–42

Fig. 7–43

Right leg
35. Right thigh (Fig. 7–41)
36. Right knee (Fig. 7–42)

37. Right shin (Fig. 7–43)

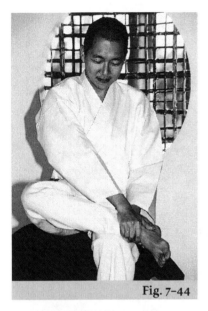

Fig. 7–44

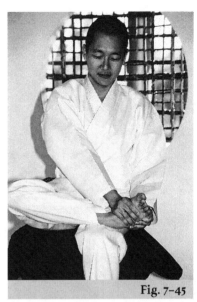

Fig. 7–45

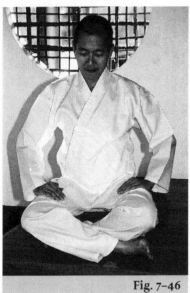

Fig. 7–46

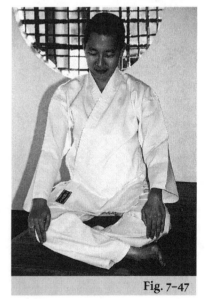

Fig. 7–47

38. Right ankle (Fig. 7–44)
39. Right foot (Fig. 7–45)

Alternative Leg Positions
40. Thighs (Fig. 7–46)
41. Knees (Fig. 7–47)

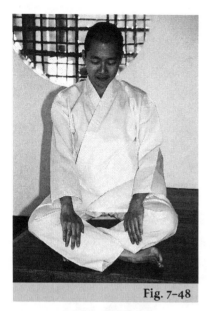

Fig. 7–48

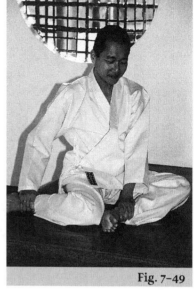

Fig. 7–49

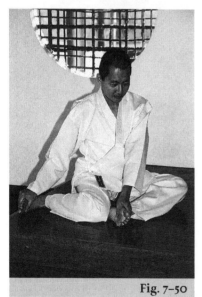

Fig. 7–50

42. Calves Fig. (7–48)
43. Ankles Fig. (7–49)
44. Tops of feet Fig. (7–50)

Head Treatment

An alternative to using the Full Body Treatment is the Head Treatment (Fig. 7–51 to Fig. 7–56) – both can be practiced from half an hour in length. Traditionally the head is the chief position to work on with *tenohira*. The head encapsulates the mind, and this mind affects the entire body at all levels. The length of time at each position will depend once again upon the sensation felt. This is especially relevant in this technique as the torso, arms and legs are worked on from a totally intuitive perspective without guiding positions. The practitioner must decide where to place the hands, the number of placements and the length of time for each.

1. The eyes and forehead (*zentô bu*) (Fig. 7–51)
2. Both temples (*sokutô bu*) (Fig. 7–52)
3. The back of the head (medulla oblongata) and forehead (*kôtô bu*) (Fig. 7–53)
4. Either side of the neck (*enzui bu*) (Fig. 7–54)
5. The crown (*tôchô bu*) (Fig. 7–55)

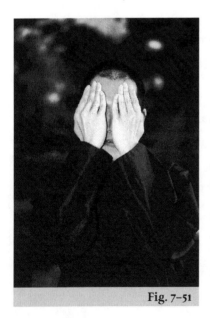

Fig. 7–51

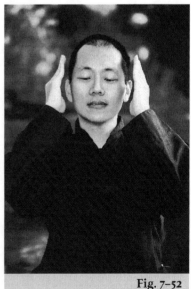

Fig. 7–52

6. After completing the head positions 1–5, the hands may be placed intuitively on the body using any of the listed Hand Poses. (Fig. 7–56)

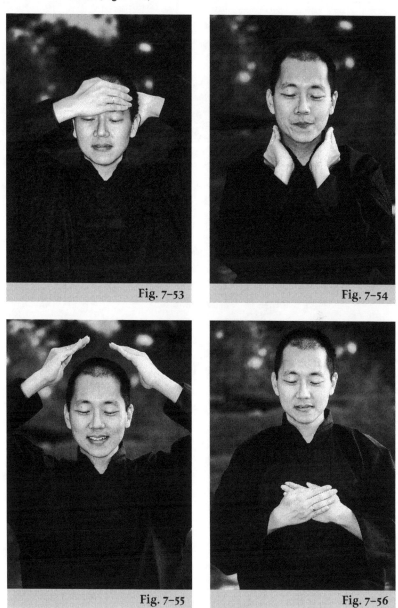

Fig. 7–53

Fig. 7–54

Fig. 7–55

Fig. 7–56

Gedoku Hô

Gedoku – detoxification
Hô – method

The *tenohira* technique, *Gedoku Hô*, uses hands placed on separate parts of the body (Hand Pose 5) and is believed to aid cleansing. This technique integrates mind and body via the hands. Historically it is known that Usui's student Hayashi taught practitioners to work on clients at both the head and *hara* at once. This concept has been replicated here for self-practice and is used in many traditional Japanese branches.

> Mind and body harmony can be thought of as self-harmony. This integration is necessarily one of the mind and body in action, a central element for mastering any classical Japanese way.[9]

Either sitting or lying, place one hand on the *hara*: connecting to your original nature. Place the other hand on the forehead: making the connection with the mind. Hold these positions for up to five minutes (Fig. 7–57). Now take your hand from your

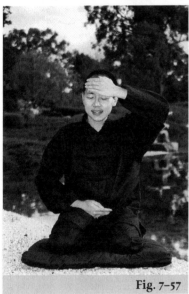

Fig. 7–57

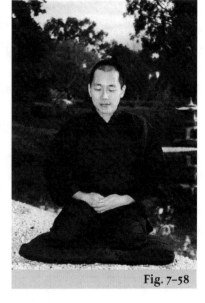

Fig. 7–58

forehead and place it over your other hand at the *hara* (Fig. 7–58). When you do this you are reminding your consciousness about your original nature. Relax quietly in this position for approximately twenty minutes.

Questions

1. Does quiet time exist in your life? How much time do you spend quietly focusing on yourself each day?
2. Do you have any physically taboo places where you feel uncomfortable placing your hands? If so, why?
3. When you place your hands on your body is there a position where you feel a strong spiritual connection?
4. Instead of needing to control the outcome of a treatment can you say to yourself, 'Whatever happens is for my best good'?
5. Do you give yourself permission to heal?

8 Jumon and Shirushi

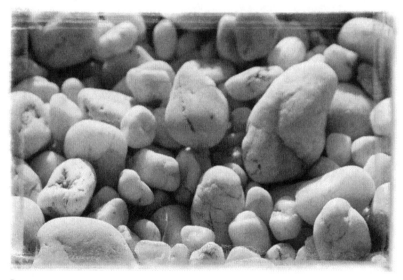

Jumon – mantras
Shirushi – symbols

Description

When one practices the system of Reiki and
moves from the first to the second level, three
symbols and mantras are taught. At the third level yet
another symbol and mantra are taught. Thus, in total,
there are four mantras and symbols taught in the system of Reiki.
Naturally, as practitioners progress through the system's three levels
new information is taught at each phase. New information is not

necessarily secret but it also is not shared until a practitioner has reached an appropriate level of understanding. This is the case with the symbols and mantras.

Basic rudiments of the system of Reiki are taught at the first level: experience with Ki work using the precepts, *kokyû* techniques and *tenohira*. Practical knowledge of these must first be gained before progressing further. With a practitioner's discipline and routine in place an environment is cultivated that extends and deepens basic knowledge of the system. *Jumon* and *Shirushi* are two tools that are used to support this objective.

To aid a practitioner's self-practice within the system; *The Japanese Art of Reiki* focuses on ways to sense your connection with the symbols and mantras. The techniques taught are designed to support your growth using these elements. The names of the mantras and the drawn symbols will not be included here. Pseudonyms have been incorporated to replace the true mantras; these aliases are CKR, SHK, HSZSN and DKM. This book does not pretend to replace a teacher or to take a practitioner through the different levels of learning – this can only occur experientially under guidance. It is instead a support and further education for those who have received the system's teachings or are interested in doing so. Do not feel left out if you have not studied any specific level of the system, as this chapter will be a valuable asset to everyone. It offers a captivating insight into where your self-practice may lead in the future.

These tools, the *jumon* and *shirushi*, are used to invoke a specific energy. Though dissimilar tools, they share this chapter as they work toward an identical aim. By using these tools you connect to certain aspects of yourself (for example Earth and Heaven Ki) and with constant practice this will awaken inner dormant energy. The realization and consciousness that these practices bring helps us to regain our full human potential. Therefore, it is not on the outside but on the inside that one should be concentrating to delve to unlimited depths. Furthermore, as one's experience develops the actual need for these tools diminishes and their energies are called upon without effort.

Source

Jumon

The Japanese name for mantra, *jumon*, means 'sound which invokes a very specific cosmic vibration'. Occasionally the mantras used in the system of Reiki have also been called *kotodama*, which means 'words carrying spirit' – clearly Shinto concepts. In ancient times, not only did the Japanese believe that the gods or *kami* were in every object and natural element, but in words too. They believed that each word uttered had the mysterious power to come true: influencing the fortunes, or misfortunes, of those who spoke and received them. The inclusion of mantras in the system of Reiki made the teachings easily accessible to Shinto practitioners.

Suzuki san states that Usui's friend and student, Eguchi Toshihiro, introduced the first three mantras CKR, SHK and HSZSN to the system. DKM with its Buddhist background is still commonly used in martial arts and Mikkyô today.

Though all four mantras are translatable, their technical meanings are less relevant than the vibrations that are invoked with their use.

Shirushi

It appears that Usui initially taught an early version of the mantras to students in the 1910s with the symbols being introduced a number of years later around 1923.[10] Both were provided to act as training wheels, which practitioners could then discard once they had 'become' the appropriate energy.[11] It would depend on a practitioner's current abilities as to which tool would be given. The symbols were provided mainly to support those who had no past energetic training – such as the naval officers to whom Usui taught a form of Ki 'first aid'.[12]

The first two symbols taught in the second level are recognizable in Japan and have Buddhist backgrounds.

The symbols have no power of their own – they act merely as a focus for a practitioner's intent. By focusing on a symbol or mantra a specific energy is stirred within the body. In traditional Japanese branches each symbol is known as a number. For example: Symbol 1, Symbol 2, Symbol 3 and Symbol 4.

The symbolism of Symbol 1 has connections to Tendai Cosmology[13] and is connected to old Japanese texts used by Tendai priests. 'Focus' is the word that the Japanese branches use to represent this symbol. By using Symbol 1, your practice will grow due to the solid foundation you create. Finding this focus and clarity of intent is a perfect introduction to the system's further depths. From a Buddhist prepective the deity that corresponds to this symbol is Daiseishi Bosatsu. This Buddha aids in awakening the wisdom within each person, leading humankind to enlightenment.

Symbol 2 can be found in the illustration of the seed syllable[14] *kiriku* and can be seen in temples across Japan. 'Harmony' is the word used by the Japanese branches to represent this symbol. After first becoming Earth Ki you then become Heaven Ki; creating harmony within the self. It is the well known Amida Nyorai (Pure Land Buddhism's main deity) who is connected to this symbol. Known as the Buddha of Infinite Light, this Buddha greets those who die and leads them to the 'Pure Land' and will not abandon even those who have committed serious transgressions. The main attributes of Amida Nyorai are to convert desire, lust and passion into the wisdom of discriminating awareness.

These first two symbols invoke correspondingly the energy of Earth and Heaven. Only when Earth and Heaven merge is there creation. In Japanese culture these elements are also represented by *in* and *yo* (popularly known as yin and yang in the Chinese culture). *In* and *yo* are body and mind, Earth and Heaven – all polar opposites. They epitomize the bringing together of two separate and contrary facets that when joined, create a whole. This is the central cosmology to the system of Reiki.

> When the Breath of Heaven and the Breath of Earth are fully integrated we have Human breath, the wellspring of our life.[15]

When Earth and Heaven energies are balanced in the body a healthy life is attained – through this balance Oneness can be experienced (Fig. 8-1).

IN	YO
Earth	Heaven
Feminine	Masculine
Left	Right
Receptive	Active
Stillness	Movement
Moon	Sun
Growing	Sowing
Shade	Light

Fig. 8-1   In & Yo Characteristics

Symbol 3 and Symbol 4 (taught respectively in Level II and Level III) are both Japanese *kanji*[16] and when read in Japanese are the actual name of the mantras HSZSN and DKM. For this reason they are not really symbols at all, but *kanji*. By working with these *kanji* you will find that your daily perceptions undergo great change.

Symbol 3 is known as 'Connection' and not for the reasons you might think. It does not connect you with anything but is instead a reminder of your innate connection to everything. Truly *knowing* this connection is different to understanding the concept literally. To begin to *know* something, the first step is the gaining and understanding of technical knowledge. It is only once you put this to practice that you then start to feel what this knowledge might mean. But you are not quite there yet – there is one more step to this process. Being It. At some point there will no longer be the separate identities of *you* and *it*. These two will become One – it is then that you truly *know* what Connection means. To become One with the universe is to *know* its rhythm and live in accordance with it. When you become aware that everything is interwoven it is easier to give yourself over to life: to let go and become One with it. The need to control and make events occur disappears. The natural evolution of a practitioner's life develops without force or suffering. Five Japanese *kanji* form this symbol (and mantra) and they can be translated into: right consciousness is the origin of everything[17]. The Buddhist deity linked to Symbol 3 is Kannon, a Bodhisattva who can hear the voices and concerns of the world and offers relief to all by changing into a multitude of different forms.

Symbol 4 is known as 'Empowerment' in Japan. The meaning of the three *kanji* that make up this word (and mantra) is 'great bright light'. Once you become this great bright light you will *know* that not only is the universe without but also within. You are in the universe and the universe is within you. Up to this point in time in *The Japanese Art of Reiki*, Oneness has been written of as the ultimate goal – but what happens when a practitioner goes further than this? This experience has no words or explanation. The great bright light is your guide to this phenomenon. Your direct experience with Symbol 4 is the embodiment of empowerment. Dainichi Nyorai, the Great Shining Buddha, is associated with this symbol and is known to shine light everywhere: giving life to and nurturing all things – leading all to a state of enlightenment.

Rewards

Humans are already enlightened – it is finding the way back to this enlightened form that is their pre-ordained journey. Though one might simply wish this to be short and easy, it is obviously not the case. For this reason visionaries, such as Usui, created systems as lights to guide one through the darkness of ignorance. *Jumon* and *shirushi* are tools to tap into one's inner knowledge. They draw you deeper into yourself but must never be totally relied upon – you must also learn to let go to allow the journey to progress deeper still.

The rewards for the *jumon* and *shirushi* are the same. These two individual tools tap into the same energy. Once you have learnt the basic understanding of Ki work in the first level of the system, you can then move on to broaden and develop that practice; learn to extend your grounded qualities, your intuitive nature and to build balance. From this place you move toward the creation of Oneness and beyond.

Today, *jumon* and *shirushi* are credited with ideals such as protection, bringing in power, enhancing, manifesting and healing karma. These were never the focus of the mantras and symbols and yet it is true some of these ideals are bi-products of their practice. There is a misunderstanding here about the basic reason for the introduction of mantras and symbols to the teachings. For example protection has been considered in the West to be a quality of Symbol 1 and CKR, and this is true, as it is a side effect of being energetically grounded. The simplicity of the truth behind these elements is unassuming and yet when used properly can profoundly affect one's existence.

Liu I Ming, a Taoist commentator from 1808 describes the pitfalls of working with symbols that might be relevant to their use in the West today: 'People of later times did not search out the meaning of the alchemical classics, but just stuck to the symbols; Confucians took them to be superstitious nonsense, while Taoists took them in a superficial manner. In extreme cases, people fixated on the symbols and arbitrarily invented all sort of practices, getting caught up in sidetracks and deviant practices.'[18]

Application

It is important to first start working with CKR and Symbol 1 and become completely aware of their functions before moving onto SHK and Symbol 2. This may take somewhere between six months and a year or even longer.

When working with either mantras or symbols it is the intent behind the ritual of chanting or visualization that creates the connection that practitioners work toward. As with any practice the set-up is vital to its ultimate success. To practice how to focus intent on the mantras and symbols, specific techniques are taught.

Using Jumon

When using *jumon* in conjunction with *shirushi* they are traditionally chanted three times. Three is considered a divine number in many cultures around the world, including Japan. Reciting *jumon* should be undertaken when one is in a quiet space (Fig. 8–2). The creation of this space sets the clear intent that you are ready to begin, thus generating a focused practice. *Jumon* invoke a specific vibration through sound. Therefore it is most effective when spoken out loud to begin with. *Jumon* must be uttered correctly as any alteration creates a different vibration

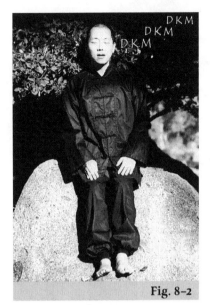

Fig. 8–2

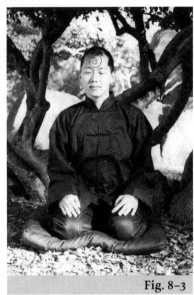

Fig. 8–3

thus producing a different manifestation. To sound the *jumon*, breathe in through the nose and vocalize out through the mouth. The source of the *Jumon* emanates from the *hara*. When you feel it is naturally time to release the breath, speak the *jumon*. The Ki filled breath, in association with the *jumon*, travels from the *hara*, expanding out through you, your mouth and your surroundings.

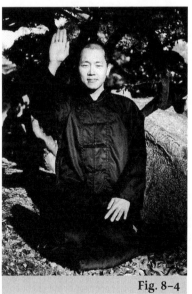

Fig. 8–4

Using Shirushi

When drawing symbols you need to keep a few aspects in mind. True knowledge of what the action is affects the quality of the outcome. The strength of this outcome is determined by your inner connection to the symbol.

If you are uncertain of what it is you are enacting then cracks will appear in which mistakes can be made. This will most likely result in a poor bonding with the symbol.

To draw a symbol various approaches can be taken:

1. Visualize drawing the symbol in the mind's eye (Fig. 8–3).
2. Physically draw with the palm of the hand (Fig. 8–4).
3. Physically draw with a finger or fingers (Fig. 8–5).

Stepping into the Ki Technique

Stand relaxed and focused with your eyes open, staring directly in front of you. Hold your palm flat and facing away from you. With the whole palm draw a Reiki symbol (Fig. 8–6). At the same time repeat the linked mantra three times. Now step into the space where you had drawn the symbol (Fig. 8–7). Remain in the energy of this space sensing the Ki. For each of the symbols and their linked mantras repeat this exercise. This will help you to sense the different energies that the mantras and symbols work with.

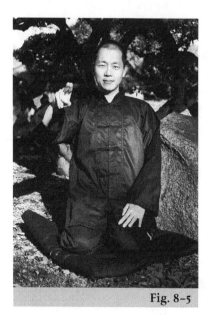

Fig. 8–5

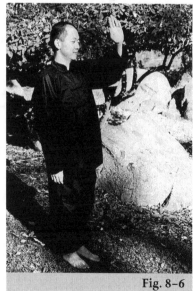

Fig. 8–6

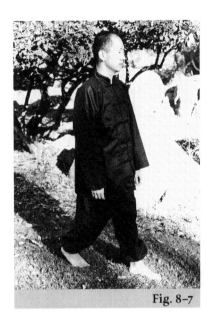

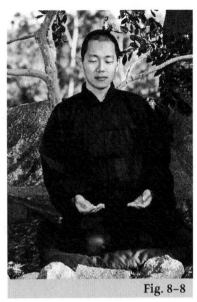

| Fig. 8–7 | Fig. 8–8 |

Jumon and Shirushi Bonding Meditation

Sit in *seiza*, focus at the ground in front of you and visualize one of the symbols. As you visualize the symbol repeat the associated mantra three times. Now sit and experience this sensation (Fig. 8–8). Do not judge it or call it names – simply be with it and see what happens. This is an excellent technique to renew your sense of connection with the *jumon* and *shirushi* (remember you are already connected). You may wish to use it with all the symbols and mantras consecutively in one go or work with one symbol at a time.

Jumon Chanting Meditation

Sit in *seiza* with your eyes gazing at the floor in front of you. Choose a mantra and chant it repeatedly. To do this: breathe in and as you breathe out vocalize the *jumon* (Fig. 8–9). Once this breath is finished just naturally allow the intake of breath into the body, bringing it down to the *hara*. As you breathe out again, the sound flows out on the waves of your breath. This becomes a mesmerizing dance of Ki, breath and sound. The activation of

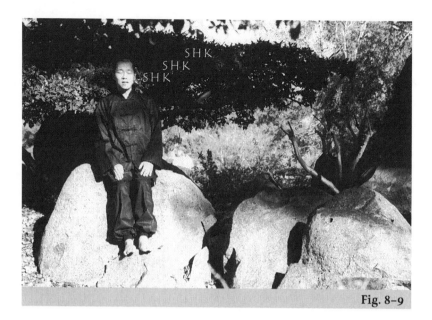

Fig. 8–9

these parts when brought together generates vibratory changes in and around you. Begin with practicing this technique for five minutes everyday, building on extending this period. After the chanting, remain seated in *seiza* and note the differences in your physical and energetic self. Continue this practice for a period of at least six months with one mantra so that you can truly gain the knowledge of how it affects you.

Questions

1. What symbols do you recognize in your life? List individual and tribal symbols – tribal symbols might be a heart (love) or a red cross (medical aid).
2. Why do you think you need symbols?
3. Do you depend on symbols or can you live without them?
4. Can a single word create change? Find examples in your life to reflect your view.
5. When you chant each mantra where do you feel it in your physical body?

9 Reiju

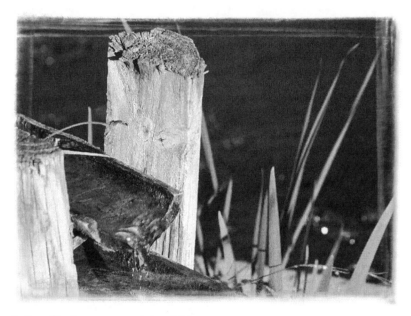

Reiju – (lit. Japanese) spiritual blessing

Description

Reiju is a ritual that is performed by a Reiki
teacher on a student and is one of the five
original elements of the system of Reiki. A student
sits in *seiza*, or on a chair, while the teacher completes a
physical and energetic ritual around him or her. The student practices
Jôshin Kokyû Hô throughout the *reiju*.

By performing *reiju* the teacher is creating a safe space for the student to draw as much Ki as he or she needs through the body. This is executed with the intent that ultimately the student will remember his or her connection to the universe. Naturally, as the student draws this Ki, the benefits related to energetic clearing will also occur.

Within the system of Reiki students must receive a minimum number of *reiju* from the teacher. The more *reiju* a student receives – the better. In traditional circles in Japan *reiju* is generally given whenever a student and teacher meet and this may be as regularly as once a week. You may receive from four *reiju* in a Reiki Level I course, three in a Level II course and one in a Level III Master/Teacher course – but this is the bare minimum. A student's graduation from one level to another is not a result of the *reiju* but, rather, it is one's personal practice that allows one to move forward. *Reiju* is seen as support for the student's journey – a blessing – rather than the crux of the entire system. The system of Reiki is so much more than *reiju* alone.

Reiju does not use symbols or mantras and is one complete ritual that does not alter with each level of the system. It remains the same – it is you the practitioner that changes.

Reiju does not give students any specific ability. The intention behind the rite is that one gets what is needed for one's personal journey – nothing more. You do not 'become attuned' to any of the levels within the system of Reiki. Ki can be channelled by anyone at anytime and therefore cannot be given or taken away from a student. This lack of intervention on a human level evidences that no one can ever come to harm with Reiki. You are an energetic being before and after *reiju* – all that you are doing is giving over to receive more of your inherited blessings. The joy of this is that it supports your journey of self-responsibility; you are always in control of what is happening with Reiki even if it is in an unconscious manner. Naturally, the more human interference in the process, the more chance there is of human weaknesses coming in to play. The responsibility placed on teachers performing *reiju* is great as they must not be tempted to manipulate, or create more out of, this ritual. Spiritual progress is therefore a must for any teacher working with *reiju*.

Chris Marsh states, 'It [*reiju*] is given in a state of mindfulness, with compassion, unconditionally without attachment to any given outcome.'

Reiju is a reminder of one's unlimited potential and this is why it is often experienced as unique. Once this instinctive memory is triggered, its recipients reel in amazement. The beauty of this potential lies within everyone and rediscovering a personal connection to it is the joy of *reiju*. It does not however give one the ability to heal, as that is an innate ability and is actually not unique at all. Developing palm-healing ability is taught and developed through the system's techniques. Other energetic methods are known to work with palm-healing, such as *Qi Gong*. The major difference between palm-healing systems is not the *reiju* but the set up of the system. If students are given a simple guideline and the confidence to do palm-healing straightway – then they can, just as is taught in the system of Reiki. Many students come to a Reiki course not because they cannot channel Ki but because they are not confident in its use at a conscious level. Once students learn the system, their intent is clear and their confidence is strong – creating successful Reiki practitioners. All that is then needed is the determination to continue to practice on the self.

The system of Reiki is popular because it offers a simple (and initially quick) structure for the awareness and development of a student's natural healing abilities supported by a teacher with *reiju*. After this early experience it is then a prerequisite that students continue to practice on themselves to generate more energy in the body and to aid in the changing of perceptions.

Source

Reiju appears to originate from Tendai Buddhism. This is not surprising as Mikao Usui was a Tendai practitioner throughout his life. *Reiju* is said to mirror a Tendai ritual called *go shimbô* that is also known as Dharma for Protecting the Body. *Go shimbô* is a purification process and is one of the first esoteric rituals that one completes in Tendai. These esoteric teachings are passed from teacher to student and are not available to the public.

It is believed that Usui performed *reiju* on his students without any physical ritual at all and simply connected to his students energetically – creating an energetic space from where Ki can be drawn. Later on students of Usui attempted to recreate this energetic ritual and found physical movements that supported the process[19].

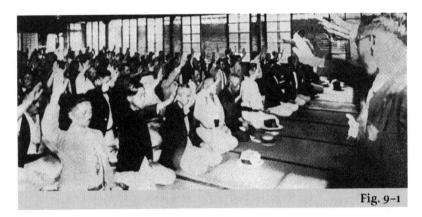

Fig. 9–1

Physical ritual has always been a tool to aid the practitioner to set clear intent. The physicality of the *reiju* continued to develop – especially once the system moved to the West where mantras and symbols were added with the hope that it would increase a teacher's ability and 'power'. This format became known as an attunement or initiation.

A famous student of Usui, Eguchi Toshihiro, is known to have also used a form of reiju called *kosho michibiki* or illuminating guidance (Fig. 9–1). This *reiju* was not performed one-on-one but rather with a group and was believed to empower participants to practice *tenohira*. Eguchi taught this at the Shiba Dojoji, which is one of the head temples of the Buddhist Pure Land sect at Shiba, Tokyo.

The true power in *reiju* is experienced when one changes direction from a physically based ritual and moves to the energetic realms. A teacher must work on one's self to the point that *reiju* can be replicated without any physical ritual at all. This simplicity is profound. If *reiju* is made more complex then more obstacles are being created for humans to address and overcome. Working solely without ritual is not advised until one has constantly practiced for many years on one's self and under the guidance of a teacher.

Rewards

The full acceptance of the *reiju* by a student can be seen as a spiritual rebirth and it is the student's choice whether to accept this potential challenge or not.

From the Lotus Sutra translated by Burton Watson:

> What falls from the cloud
> Is water of a single flavor,
> But the plants and trees, thickets and groves,
> Each accept the moisture that is appropriate to its portion. [20]

To receive *reiju* is to quench one's thirst for spiritual connection. Many factors affect the *reiju* experience. One important factor is the student's trust in the teacher. For this reason it is integral to get to know or feel connected to your teacher prior to a course. When one is relaxed and comfortable receiving *reiju* – more Ki can be drawn through the body. If one is uptight and defensive it is unlikely that much Ki will be acquired. The state of mind is therefore a factor that will affect the process and the outcome.

To define why each *reiju* experience is different would be asking for human rationalization. As with every aspect of the system of Reiki it is imperative that one lets go and accepts the outcome for what it is. All that can be known is that the more self-practice undertaken, the greater the self-knowledge and inner understanding gained. Letting go is a task and benefit simultaneously.

When students and teachers practice regularly on themselves, more Ki can be channeled through the body. This is due to the energetic pathways becoming stronger. Consequently, in every day life you will naturally be stronger and your ability to help yourself and others will drastically increase. By receiving repeated *reiju* the students enhance their own energy levels. The teacher is merely a channel for the energy to move through. Though this is true – the more the teacher energetically evolves, the higher the teacher's vibration level and the more energy that is channeled. This also supports the notion that the teacher does not have any special 'power' over the students – personal development is up to the student and the amount of work that the student completes.

Application

To perform reiju is not about re-enacting a ritual; anybody can memorize the physical

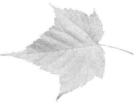

moves of *reiju* within an hour. The strength of the *reiju* is, in fact, not in the ritual itself but in the teacher's state of mind. If the *reiju* is performed in the right state of mind then the student will receive the most benefit from it. In Usui's time, students would learn *reiju* very late on in the extended teachings. Until then it is said he believed the possibility of understanding the depth of Ki connection could not be fully understood.

To set this state of mind, a teacher needs to focus awareness on the connection within one's self, the energy in the room, the student and most importantly where one fits in on a universal level. Never forget that it is even possible to go beyond the concept of *reiju* as a ritual – with personal practice.

A significant aspect of a teacher's self-practice is developing this connection. There are various ways to do this. Following are two Japanese preparations that you may choose from. Why not practice both and find the one that helps you connect most to your inner core. This can be a practice in itself or be followed up by the performing of *reiju*. If there is no one for you to practice *reiju* on after your preparation then be creative and perform it on a chair. You may even wish to sit in the chair afterwards to receive the blessing. After all, it is the intent that matters.

Reiju Preparation 1

Before beginning the preparation observe the cleansing routine of *Kenyoku Hô*. Prior to this, remember to always practice the six principles for preparation: know your technique, stand with your eyes focused out in front, release all tension from the body, bring the mental focus to the *hara*, and allow the hands to rise in *gasshô*.

Bring both hands down and place them one on top

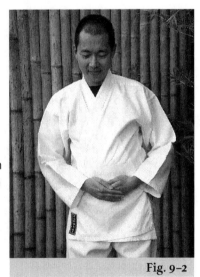

Fig. 9–2

of the other at the *hara* (Fig. 9–2). At the same time consciously focus your mind on the *hara* – you are now integrating the mind and body. Sense the balance this creates within your being and focus on DKM until you feel a strong connection.

To close off, bring the hands back up into the *gasshô* position.

Reiju Preparation 2

As with the first preparation technique complete the cleansing routine of *Kenyoku Hô*. Prior to this remember to always practice the six principles for preparation: know your technique, stand with your eyes focused out in front, release all tension from the body, bring the mental focus to the *hara* and allow the hands to rise in *gasshô*. Keep you mind focused on the *hara,* throughout this preparation. This is your Ki connection.

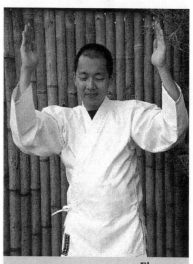

Fig. 9–3

Hold your arms in a v-shape next to your head and out to the side of the body with your palms facing upwards (Fig. 9–3). Experience the sensation of Ki moving down through your head and arms, moving down through you and clearing the body. Turn your palms toward the earth and lower your arms out to the side (Fig. 9–4) until they come together in front of the *hara*. Now put your left hand into your right hand with your thumbs touching

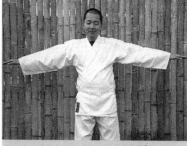

Fig. 9–4

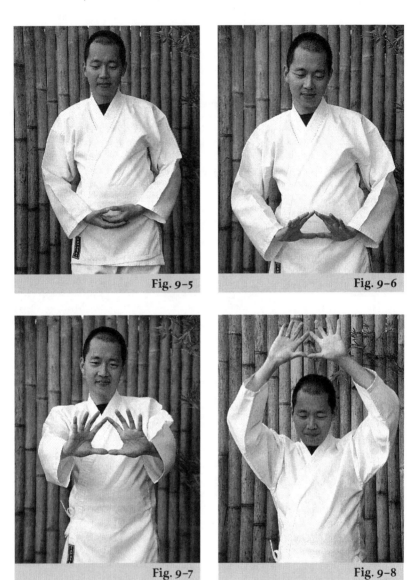

Fig. 9–5

Fig. 9–6

Fig. 9–7

Fig. 9–8

lightly (Fig. 9–5). Sense the Ki radiating from your *hara*.

With your hands, create the sun mudra (*nichirin in*) and move your hands from your *hara* (Fig. 9–6) in a circular movement out in front of the body (Fig. 9–7) and up until they are above your head (Fig. 9–8). Now open your hands and bring them out to the side

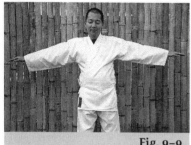

Fig. 9–9

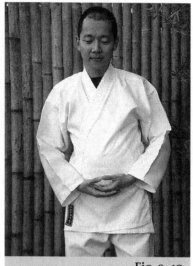

Fig. 9–10

(Fig. 9–9) and back down to in front of the *hara* (Fig. 9–10). Repeat moving your hands in the sun mudra position up to the head and down to the *hara* two more times.

Once you are finished bring your hands into *gasshô* and begin the *reiju*.

Questions

Think of a time in your life when you felt totally aligned with your existence, when everything went right and you were amazed at your 'good luck'.

1. Why do you think this occurred?
2. Why did it change?
3. What changes could you make in your life right now to bring back that sense of alignment?

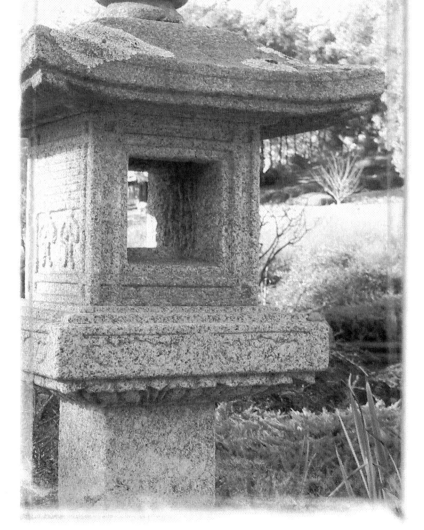

Part III
Practicing Reiki

10 Choosing a Reiki Course

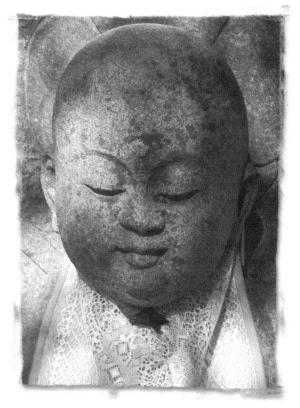

Once you have decided to begin studying the system of Reiki, a course needs to be chosen. The most important factors affecting your choice of course will most probably be what is being taught and who is teaching.

The Course

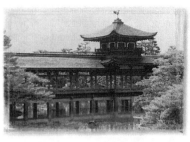

For those interested in learning Japanese based teachings there are certain lineages to look for: these most likely comprise elements of what is taught in *The Japanese Art of Reiki*. A lineage is the line that is traced back through one's teacher to the founder of the system. No two teachers are alike as are no two courses and therefore it is impossible to state exactly who teaches what. When you study in a certain lineage you are never assured of a specific standard or information. Currently, there are no safeguards protecting you and it is your responsibility alone to choose wisely. Research (such as reading this book and *The Reiki Sourcebook*) will put you in good stead to have a solid understanding to direct questions from.

Here are some lineages that date from Usui and are Japanese based and are taught to students in the West:

> *Usui Reiki Ryôhô*
> Usui Mikao – Taketomi Kanichi – Koyama Kimiko – Doi Hiroshi
>
> *Komyo Reiki Kai*
> Usui Mikao – Hayashi Chûjirô – Yamaguchi Chiyoko – Hyakuten Inamoto
>
> *Gendai Reiki Hô* (fusion between Japan and West)
> Usui Mikao – Taketomi Kanichi – Koyama Kimiko – Doi Hiroshi
>
> *Jikiden Reiki*
> Usui Mikao – Hayashi Chûjirô – Yamaguchi Chiyoko – Yamaguchi Tadao

There are a certain number of key levels taught in the Japanese system of Reiki today. This is generally three, though in some lineages either the second or third levels are divided up into two parts: creating four levels in total. Each level is taught with a break in between as at each level the student learns new techniques for developing Ki work and must become proficient in these before moving on to study further.

Most levels of the system of Reiki today are taught first in an intensive course with follow-up training occurring after the intensive is finished. The reason for this is that receipt of a certificate (generally received at the end of the intensive) indicates that you are now beginning that level rather than completing it. As you are a beginner it is then expected that the real work should begin for you to be able to progress to enter into the next level.

To fully understand the system of Reiki a prospective practitioner must first look at why he or she wants to learn it in the first place. There are a number of avenues that can be taken. For example: you can complete a weekend course, or you can complete a weekend course *and* practice once a week on yourself at a practice evening, or you can complete a weekend course *and* attend a weekly practice evening *and* incorporate a daily personal routine.

By just completing a weekend course some change can be expected along with a certain understanding of the system. Naturally the more you practice, the deeper the levels of change and understanding that will be accessed. So within the system of Reiki there are different levels a practitioner can delve into, depending on his or her involvement.

To become proficient in anything one must practice and for this a supportive course is of the essence. Support can come in many shapes and sizes. It is of importance that a teacher be available to discuss a student's technical and spiritual growth. Reiki practitioners around the world today often come together to practice palm-healing on one another – this wonderful support can be developed to be much more effective. The Japanese way is that Reiki should be an ongoing study and practice groups can therefore be an extension of a Reiki course with the same five elements being practiced and discussed rather than just a 'sharing' of energy. In this way a student's learning is encouraged and developed. Surely you would like to know that what you are doing is correct and that your practice has not derailed at some point? Attendance at a regular practice group is very beneficial energetically to a student also – even though one may be working solely on the self. There are similarities here with attending the gym or practicing aerobics – you could just as well jump up and down at home to get fit but you do not. Instead you make an appointment, go to a class and work on yourself within a group environment. This routine supports you in your personal practice and just by aligning yourself with others and sharing the same motivation you are spurred on to work harder and achieve your goals. The teacher also performs *reiju* at these practice groups to offer you not only motivational but spiritual support. Weekly Reiki practice groups and regular retreats are consequently an excellent way to continue your practice with the support of your teacher and peers.

Underpinning the practice of Reiki are many Japanese concepts and philosophies. A course that claims to be 'traditional' must therefore include these components. Western systems inevitably teach New Age movement influenced teachings such as the chakra system.

The price of a course is an issue for many. Course costs should be reliant on the teacher's valuation of the course set-up. You should therefore be paying for your teacher's education and experience, the course venue and associated costs, practical course materials like manuals and the level of support systems offered after the course. One cannot, and does not, pay for the Ki itself – that is beyond our human control. When choosing a course be aware of *all* costs that you will be asked to incur and do not fall into the trap of paying for a cheap and 'easy' first level course only to be asked to pay thousands for a rising number of levels (today some western branches have seven or more levels). Lastly, always make sure you know where you stand as far as refund policies go.

When you begin a course, though you may have currently no intention to do a second or third level course, just imagine that you will be continuing on to these levels. Is this the course that you will get the most out of? It is great to educate yourself with different teachers but it is difficult and sometimes confusing to come in half way through a course's training. For this reason it is best to begin from the first level again when you decide to take another Reiki course. Occasionally there are also special 'catch-up' courses available for those who have trained elsewhere. The first level of the system of Reiki is the most important as it puts the whole system and how it is taught into context.

Choosing a Reiki Course

When looking for a course in a Japanese system search for one that:

- Offers Japanese lineages such as those listed here.
- Teaches three or four major levels (sometimes four are taught when either the second or third level are divided into two sub sections).
- Requires that students develop energetically between each level.
- Teaches each level at the time that is appropriate to a student's level of experience.
- Works with the Japanese energetic system and techniques rather than the New Age chakra system or techniques.
- Offers ongoing support and the opportunity to upgrade knowledge and experience (perhaps through weekly practice groups and retreats).
- Is open about all costs that are to be paid by a student for all levels.
- A student is happy to continue through to all levels with.

The Teacher

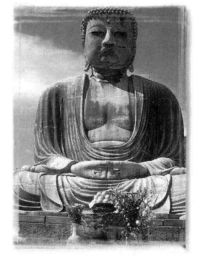

To begin with, a student has every right to ask for a teacher's lineage. This will indicate if the teachings are Japanese in nature, however there are more questions to be asked before you make any further decisions. A prospective student needs to divine whether the teacher is an ethical, knowledgeable and trustworthy individual. Though the system of Reiki is not a transmission system (as practiced in Tibetan Buddhism) you are naturally affected by how and what your teacher teaches. What you eventually practice will be a reflection of these teachings. Some teachers instruct in other forms of energetic healing – find out what they are and if they are aligned with what you are looking for. It is disappointing if you find a teacher that puts on one hat for the Japanese system of Reiki and then another hat for a system of Reiki that has a different history and understanding of energy. This signals a lack of integration of the system into the teacher's life.

Traditionally, the role of a teacher is to guide a student through all the practices involved with each level. This aids the student in trusting the process and learning to let go, as a result experiencing each element at its fullest. Confidence is gained when tuition is knowledgeable and clear. Thus the teacher's assuredness ensures the level of clarity of intent for the student's own practice. This does not mean that a teacher supplies a student with all the answers – that is an impersonation of teaching – but that a student is guided to find the answers: becoming empowered.

Your teacher's own journey is important to the extent that you should 'travel' spiritually with him or her as a student. If one's teacher does not have a personal routine of self practice then there is no point in learning from them. Some teachers believe that their effort in healing or helping others qualifies them as good Reiki teachers. It may make them 'good' people and energetically benefit their self practice to some degree but it is not self practice itself. Working with others is an excellent activity but it can be deceiving. Many teachers and practitioners get hooked on receiving gratifying responses from those they have helped or 'wowed' with 'their' Reiki. Personal practice is mostly about hard work and at times not gratifying whatsoever but it is true self-development. As a potential student you will want to find out that your teacher practices what he or she preaches. If a teacher asserts no need for self practice then you must quickly move on – it is only an enlightened soul that needs no practice and an enlightened soul has no need for claims of illumination. A student must give and receive respect and have a sense that during one's evolution trust will grow and blossom.

There is an initial phase where you may feel bedazzled when reminded of your true nature – your Ki connection. It is all too easy to credit a teacher with this awe while it should be directed at your own amazing self. If a teacher misunderstands these energetic fundamentals then he or she may believe that they have miraculously gained a supernatural power and can 'do' things to others. This concept unfortunately places the 'power' in your teacher's hands and renders you unempowered. You become controlled by your teacher's 'ability' and consequently you see no need to practice. In such a situation you may also notice that, as times goes by, the 'wow' factor decreases and decreases and suddenly you are left with just a vague memory of what this connection had meant. So many students of Western forms of Reiki complain of this and wish to be 're-attuned' – not realizing that they were never attuned to anything in the first place. It is not the attunement that reminds them of who they are but their own efforts.

A teacher's attitude to others is an indication that they understand and practice what is taught in the system of Reiki. If this is the case the teacher will never make claims to be 'energetically stronger' or 'more powerful' than any another system or teacher. This is bravado and false advertising and has no place within the system of Reiki. Naturally there will be different qualities in the technical elements of courses themselves (some are better than others) but it is impossible to say that 'my' energy is better than 'yours'. Reiki is the energy of everything and therefore cannot be compared to be stronger or weaker than anything. If you do come across someone insisting that their energy is 'better' then ask them to prove it to you – they cannot. Be wary though as the mind is much stronger than you may think. If someone says to you, ' You are now going to feel a vibrant energy' it is more than likely that you do. Once a thought is implanted in you it can be difficult to think otherwise. Some people are also overwhelmed by the supposed abilities of others that they let themselves be swayed by this. These people may agree with the claim simply to make themselves look knowledgeable and to appear energetically skilled. Ki work is subjective and the interpretation of it is reliant on each individual situation.

A teacher must never hold onto students as if they were showpieces in a menagerie. This is where respect for a teacher and respect for a student is reciprocated through a shared journey. For a time they may travel together but then there may come a time to part. A teacher shall not judge a student's choice of further training knowing that the student has his or her own path to take. No credit, either, may be taken for a student's growth, as this was ultimately the student's task and success.

One last important aspect to choosing the right course is to look at a teacher's Code of Ethics and Code of Practice. Is there one? A Code of Ethics outlines how a teacher agrees to deal with you as a student, his or her peers and the community at large. The Code of Practice offers a guideline of the teacher's business practices. Today, even if you are studying a Japanese form of the system of Reiki, you will find that most teachers are members of an association. An association will set a minimum standard that the teacher must conform to (or no longer remains a member) and often has a set Code of Ethics and Code of Practice that members work under. There is an element of safety knowing that your teacher is a member of a respected association and that the teacher's activities fall under its codes.

Choosing a Reiki Teacher

When searching for a teacher, take into consideration the teacher's:

- Lineage.
- Understanding of Ki work.
- Understanding of the Japanese culture and history of the system of Reiki.
- Personal spiritual journey and your connection to it.
- Support for a student's personal development through providing one-on-one contact where necessary.
- Talent in allowing students to find out the answers for themselves.
- Ability to practice the spiritual elements of the system without needing to 'manipulate' the energy.
- Capacity to 'let go' – rather than create more complex rituals.
- Claims – that they are realistic and verifiable rather than ego orientated. That no unsubstantiated statements are made about the system or a teacher's personal Ki work.
- Respect for past and present students – noting that no judgments about others are made.
- Ownership of a Code of Ethics and Code of Practice and membership in an association.
- Ability to inspire you!

Meet with a teacher and after looking at all these issues concerning both the course and the teacher trust your gut reaction. If you feel good, then do it – you are sure to learn something. If you are uncertain, take time – there is no rush. The right teacher and course will appear. Know what it is you are looking for and always make sure that your choice addresses these priorities.

11 Developing a Regular Routine

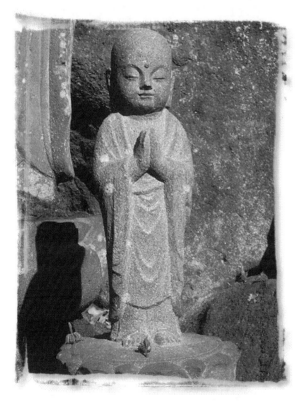

The word 'routine' conjures up a love/hate sensation in most people. Though humans function best when using routine, just thinking about 'knuckling down' can be a real turn-off – and this is before you even begin. In fact, it is often those initial first steps that seem the hardest.

The Living Practice

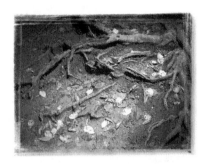

To make the transition to becoming a regular practitioner as easy as possible one must be well organized and prepared and this is part of what routine can offer. With a good clear structure, your practice can be turned into a natural part of your existence instead of a task that must be tackled – this is called a living practice.

Your day is already divided up into all sorts of routines. These have been incorporated into your life at various stages either consciously or unconsciously. They are simple things like: how you dress, shower and eat. You do not mind doing these things (though you may have initially as a child), as they are now an integrated part of your every day life.

There are other less obvious routines in your life too. Take note, for example, of *how* you think about things. Believe it or not you have taught yourself specific ways to think and act and walk and talk. These, too, are your own personal routines.

Humans continue to repeat their routines even though some may be damaging to their health and happiness.

Do you have a routine that whenever something unpleasant happens, you go and buy the biggest bar of chocolate you can find and the strongest, sweetest, frothiest cappuccino and ... over indulge? Or do you drink till you forget or shop till you credit card screams 'No More!' You put these routines in place.

Having been the creator of these routines suggests that you also have the power to be their destroyer. The choice is now yours to create new routines – consciously. By setting up a personal spiritual practice this is what you are doing. In the short term this in itself might be disruptive but the long-term benefits of conscious living are exceptional.

Choosing consciously to create new routines is choosing to live a life working toward spiritual growth. There are just two paths here – toward or away from spiritual growth – and you are constantly walking down one of them. Every action you take affirms the path that you are setting for yourself. Therefore, this decision to begin a routine is a conscious affirmation of your spiritual aims. It needs to be taken seriously and might be the toughest part of the whole routine process for you.

In the effort to follow through with your routine it must not be separated from every day life. Life today is generally compartmentalized into work, play and practice. Combining all three activities is the most effective tool that will bring about spiritual progress. If you are focusing on compassion during your routine, for example, and yet treating those at work or home with disdain or contempt – then you achieve little. A rounded routine, as is suggested by the system of Reiki, brings focus to the many aspects of everyday life through its five elements. Initially, one's practice feels detached but over time it will flow into daily living.

To be able to call yourself a practitioner it is imperative that you practice on yourself daily. This does not mean to hop into bed, put your hands on your stomach and fall asleep but rather follow a regular routine. It is easy to just sit back and think that it *will* all happen automatically, but nothing ever happened that way. The more a practitioner puts in, the more a practitioner receives in return.

Creating a Routine

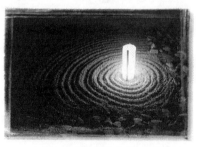

Routine, too, is a form of ritual. Ritual energetically activates three essential components – the three diamonds of body, mind and heart. When these pull together as One, balance is created and working towards one's goal becomes effortless. With the physical body grounded in the practice and the mind knowing what to do, the spirit is freed to soar with the practice.

As you read through this book you may think, 'Yes, I can do this. I'm going to do three hours practice everyday and then in about one years time my life will be totally different.' Wouldn't that be great? It would – but it is also highly unlikely as three hours a day is a great deal to ask of your self. You have set the challenge too high and after a week you do not even want to hear the word 'practice' again. This is often due to the guilt you feel at having procrastinated – you have not followed through with the spontaneous promise to yourself.

There will be many challenges along this path. How many excuses can you think of not to do your practice? Do not worry; you are not alone. This is the constant challenge of each practitioner and not one can honestly say they have totally resisted temptation. The sparkling red apple glistens in the wings waiting to capture your attention. The best way to deal with this is to create a functional and realistic daily routine.

Time is initially a crucial part of your routine. Find out how much time you have in a day to work on yourself and how many times you would like to do this. You may have half an hour in the morning and half an hour in the evening. You may be a shift worker and can fit in an hour after lunch or perhaps as a beginner you believe you can only set aside fifteen minutes a day. It is okay. It is better to do some rather than none. If one day you do not have the time, then at the appointed practice time just pause, take a moment's notice of your breath, go inside and center yourself through your *hara*. You have upheld your contract with yourself and are well on the way to developing a living practice.

Once you begin your practice at your allotted time it is also important that you continue it. You may practice for a number of months, have a brief holiday where you forget to practice, and later take it up again. This is not the best form of practice. Consistency creates a moving, living practice. For this reason, too, it is better to choose an amount of time convenient for you.

To help develop a routine choose a special practice area. Very few people have the luxury of a meditation room or large space that they can call their own. For this reason choosing a perfect place for your practice will need to take into account a number of things.

Most importantly find somewhere where you are not in the way of others. Do not bother to try to get everyone to stay away from you as it is far easier to keep away from them. Therefore, your timing will have to take into account the actions of others and, as with the attention to timing, keep the venue regular.

The space you choose may be small and may even double as something else when it is not in use as your practice area. Imagine though that this space is yours and imbue it with the respect that should be accorded to a sacred venue. This establishes a special atmosphere for you when you practice, allowing you to move effortlessly into your inner space.

Quiet is not the absolute prerequisite you might think it is. It is helpful but noise does not signify that your practice should be disturbed. Sound is a natural part of human life and oversensitivity to noise is your mind looking for distraction from your practice.

Ritual helps to focus the mind and therefore routine will stop the mind from wandering in your practice. Having a set time of day and a set place to practice in, assures you that these elements will not be diverting you from commencing your practice.

The 21–Day Program

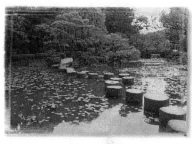

Naturally, ongoing practice is the highest form of training. Various routines can support you in this. A practical routine is the concept of a twenty-one day program – this gives a practitioner a beginning to work from and a goal to work toward. It is taught as a pre-cursor to ongoing daily work and governs the practitioner's practice carefully. If a practitioner can stick with the process for twenty-one days then a solid grounding is created for the practitioner to develop his or her practice from.

This concept is a traditional one in Japan and is found in forms such as Shugendô and Tendai. For example; traditional meditations, like the Buddhist *hokkesen*, are practiced for the duration of twenty-one days.

The twenty-one-day practice is generally commenced immediately after an initial Reiki course. It does not matter which level the student has completed, as it is a valid technique for all three levels. In fact a practitioner desiring to intensively clear the body, mind and heart can initiate a program such as this at any time. Throughout life, shifts continue to attempt to take place. This is virtually a never-ending process. By using this program you can find a way to work through them. It can relieve you from repeatedly hitting up against the same issues time and time again not quite completing these Ki shifts. Once you have moved through the shifts you begin to understand better how to deal with them with this ongoing task becoming less of a struggle and more of a creative flight.

Following is a suggested outline for a practitioner's twenty-one-day program that you can adjust to your own circumstances (Fig. 11 – 1). There are four individual routines and some may be practiced consecutively or at separate times of the day. The length of each routine in this practice is reliant on the experience of the practitioner and the situation.

The program includes techniques from Part II of *The Japanese Art of Reiki* as well as the task of writing a daily page. It can be difficult to express yourself as change transpires and writing is an excellent outlet. You can write about daily events, raging emotions, your practice and anything that takes your attention. Do not judge it; do not even re-read it for the moment – just let it come out. Fear, anger, grief, relief, exultation and love all pour out as the Ki flows freer. Paper soaks up these feelings. Take a sheet and sop up the emotional remains of experience. As with every other routine in this program it must be performed regularly. There is no point in doing it if the commitment is not true. For those days where you do not know what to write or do not want to write, just write exactly that. It may stimulate you to continue writing on another subject. *What* you write is not important – *that* you write, is.

Due to the intensity of this twenty-one-day program, by its finish a shift in a practitioner's Ki will most likely have taken place. Obviously Level II or III practitioner's will have to decide which techniques they prefer to work on in their allotted timeslots and must remember not to overdo it. Make your routine powerful yet practical and keep in mind that it is just for twenty-one days.

A major advantage in this practice being for just twenty-one days is that by the end of it, having felt shifts and gained new insights, you are more than stimulated to continue practicing on yourself. You will then take from your routine the elements that you wish to continue working with on a daily basis. No longer will you need to set a number of days or weeks to work with but you will be happy to settle down on the incredible path of spiritual growth.

Begin each routine with the six principles to ready yourself for practice: decide upon the technique/s, sit or stand, softly gaze with the eyes, release all tension from the body, bring the mental focus to the *hara*, and allow the hands to rise in *gasshô*.

Routine	The Practice and Level	Page No.	Length of Practice	Regularity of Practice
Routine 1. *Gokai*	**Level I, II & III** Chant the entire precepts (this may be replaced by another *gokai* technique).	p.71	Three times consecutively.	In the morning and evening.
Routine 2. **Techniques**	**Level I, II & III** *Kenyoku Hô* followed by *Jôshin Kokyû Hô* and/or *Seishin Toitsu*. **Level II & III** *Jumon* and *Shirushi* techniques. **Level III** *Reiju* preparation and practice.	p.80 p.85 p.87 p.127 p.137	**Level I** Begin with 15 minutes in total and work toward half an hour over the three weeks. **Level II & III** Begin with 30 minutes in total and work toward an hour over the three weeks.	Once a day.
Routine 3. *Tenohira*	**Level I** Full Body Treatment. **Level II & III** Head Treatment and/or *Gedoku Hô*.	p.104 p.116 p.118	Approximately half an hour a day and may be practiced lying down or seated.	Once a day.
Routine 4. **Writing**	**Level I, II & III** Keep a daily diary.	p.160	Write a page minimum per day.	Once a day.

Fig. 11–1   The 21 – Day Program

Another way to teach concentration on your practice is to practice for a certain number of days and then have one day free, continuing in an ongoing cycle. Make this complete cycle an even number of days and you will find that it requires determination and focus to retain the cycle. This routine will aid your concentration and determination levels by distracting the mind from making excuses not to practice – you are too busy counting the days.

Clearing

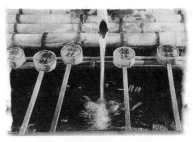

Changes that take place during Ki work are recognized as being of a clearing nature. This is where the body, mind and heart release their attachments. You are not detaching from life – you are actually letting go of the baggage you will not need on your journey. This might be attachment to other's beliefs or your own distracting habits.

The best way to aid healing of the body, mind and heart is to work with a system such as Reiki. Improving the flow of Ki indicates that energy is being forged through the three diamonds to places where it may previously have laid stagnant. When this stagnant Ki moves, the body reacts. These reactions are what we know as ill health. Today, ill heath is considered something that needs to be avoided at all costs. Yet, with the body having its own inbuilt healing system there are other ways to view this phenomenon. Why does the body get sick in the first place? Generally because it has taken something on that it needs to get rid of. It is this 'ridding' process that results in the symptoms that are called ill health. When your body needs to move something you call yourself sick and yet it is simply the body doing the right and natural thing to protect itself. If it did not react, the physical body would have been dead long ago. So this process should not be stopped or messed with. If anything, it needs to be encouraged.

A clearing can range from a cold to physical pain to emotional imbalance. After being stagnant for a time, the sensation of stagnant Ki reminds the body that it has stopped something away. The body attempts to continue the clearing process, to return itself back to a naturally balanced state. Perhaps there are many issues related to this stagnant energy and one by one the moving Ki nudges them loose. Your body knows what it has to do and all you have to do is support it in that process and that is what Reiki is for.

Though a clearing may not sound like a bunch of laughs it is a most natural and positive experience. Seen from this viewpoint, a practitioner is actually grateful for illness in the knowledge that the body is working away at shifting energy so that he or she may move on to a new and healthier level.

Sometimes that level is never reached. A practitioner may resist the clearing to the point that it returns to its stagnant state – only to rear its head again later. A practitioner may pass from this world while in a state of clearing – this is true for anyone who dies of ill health. Herein lies the joy and pain of our human experience.

When you begin to work with Reiki you will notice clearing taking place. At first, you think, 'oh no I've caught the flu that's going around,' – but it is not. This is your body doing its best to flow with you in your 'making whole' process. Do not rush for the anti-histamines or aspirins, continue your routine and watch yourself move through it with ease.

There might also be a reaction that says, 'oh no I've taken the wrong road and I really don't like what has come up now,' – but it is okay. The most wonderful part about this clearing is that at some level you are in control. So, though you may feel way out of control, you have opened yourself up to heal to such an extent that the Ki is flowing thick and fast, jostling everything out of the way. To experience such a reaction you are most likely the type of person who throws him- or herself headfirst into a situation. Did you say to yourself, 'I am going to heal no matter what'? If you did – you asked for it. You are not a 'victim' to the energy. You make choices and in the same way that you have thrown yourself in deep, you can pull yourself back out. This path is in your hands. If it becomes too much, pull back, practice less or stop altogether as you re-assess your situation. No one should put themselves in a position where they feel they can no longer handle it and everyone must remember that there is no ulterior force at work here – there is just you and you are in control. Take your power.

Another reaction you might have is, 'wow, I feel amazing,' – and you do. Your task is to retain that sense of wonderment – that fresh, baby faced view and observe. Through this detachment judgments are not made, dramas are not enacted, and openness is a natural state.

Judging is non-acceptance. A very young child does not judge its toys. It does not have a 'favorite' as you might be lead to believe. Favoritism only comes about in a child's mind from being asked, 'Which is your favorite?' – the concept is initially foreign. The child may be attracted to a certain look or sensation in a toy but it does not judge the toy for that. This does not make it a 'good' or 'bad' toy – it simply is, at this exact moment, the toy the child is playing with.

By paying attention to all emotions, a practitioner can become an observer rather than an active participant in the drama of daily life. Drama is addictive and to unlearn it is an enormous charge. Supported by the daily practice of Ki work, a practitioner can begin to differentiate between drama and healthy living. This frees a practitioner to experience true feelings in a natural and spontaneous manner.

12 Self-healing, a Way of Life

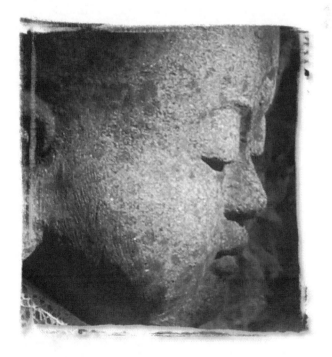

To self-heal is to take responsibility for everything that happens to you at all levels: body, mind and heart.

This sounds like an enormous task but to self-heal is an inborn ability. Humans enter this world with the gifts to help them develop and grow spiritually: to 'make whole'. So, it is up to you how you utilize these gifts.

Your Courage

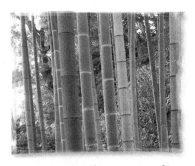

The community that surrounds you may not necessarily support your natural self-healing skills. As a child you may not have been made aware that you are an energetic being – one that deserves respect and support.

A child will learn what it needs to survive in the surroundings that it grows up in. Some of these survival skills may not support self-healing and in fact may even suppress them. If a child does not see others purposefully using their self-healing abilities then there is also no stimulus to develop them.

For these reasons, your practice is a role model to the rest of the world. Begin self-healing and then watch it affect every single being you encounter. You automatically heal others without even physically working on them. Becoming more comfortable with yourself relaxes you, making you friendlier and less fearful. This outlook affects your colleagues, your partner, even the people you meet in the supermarket. It reminds them of the joy that a fearless life can bring. Exposure to courageous living brings about a domino effect of lit up smiling faces.

Your World

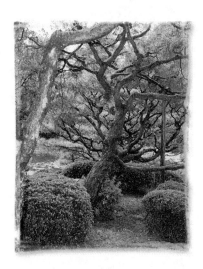

Do not become a recluse hiding away from the world because it is so messed up and you do not want to 'catch' it. It is not catching unless you let it be. Do find your space in the world. A place where you are content and can practice your daily routine in relative peace. Contentment means feeling secure and safe in your environment – physically, financially and socially.

An integral part of respecting yourself is to live a healthy life. The word healthy has surely been around the block and back in the last couple of years. There is an acknowledgement that healthy is good but the advertising gurus keep changing its meaning. Healthy living is relative to your experience. You know what is healthy for you. You know what makes you feel light and full of energy.

Firstly, to gauge if you are living a healthy life look at the energy that you are taking into your body. Your eating habits are extremely important in this. To find out whether you eat well check how you feel *after* you have eaten the food. Physically, the food you eat must nourish and cleanse you – not deposit toxins in the body. It must support you in your aim to live a balanced and mobile life, physically and energetically. Water, too, is a natural resource that assists humanity with clearing. Coffee may no longer attract you when you begin Ki work. Drink water, lots of it, at room temperature so that it does not shock your system with extremes of heat or cold – it feels so good. Together with food, these forms of energy bring health and aid in the removal of unwanted waste.

Your environment acts on you from the outside too. A large percentage of humans are working in jobs that they hate and with people they cannot connect to. The effect on the body of having to struggle constantly with this situation, five days out of seven, is an enormous strain. It drains your energy and leaves you in recovery mode throughout most of your 'free' time. The bottom line here is the issue of 'free' and 'not free' time. To divide our lives up into these categories is like saying there is a time to live and a time not to live. To claim good health – you need to be alive. This problem is partially a community one and partially your own. Humans have set communities up to function in this manner – separating a time for play from a time for work. You have the choice to join this mentality and support it or you can buck the system and create your own experience. This does not mean to immediately quit your job and take up selling jewelry on the corner. Within the boundaries that exist in your working life you can make change. Remember, by building your inner energy you can develop an internal strength that is not so easily swayed by your environment. This inner core can give you a new perspective on your work. Eventually, you may wish to move onto something that is more satisfying for you and it may not offer great amounts of money or status but it could give you your life back.

The same can be said about friends. Change can really scare friends. They may be so used to sitting down with you and having a 'good' gossip or getting drunk, that if you decide not to partake in these activities due to a more conscious outlook – you may no longer be considered 'fun'. Fortunately, your new perspective on life may alter what *you* consider fun as you find more appropriate ways to know joy. Not all friends will follow through with you on your journey. How you treat yourself and others in general alters with Ki work as you begin to live less destructively – cultivating Ki rather than losing it.

Even your home environment may change. An apartment in the inner city might evolve into a house in the country. If not, perhaps you may look for ways to escape by taking regular breaks from your busy surroundings to go for a quiet walk in the forest, to sit next to a waterfall or to listen to the waves on a secluded beach.

Pleasure is gifted to you from a world that some may no longer be able to see. As a baby you touched it and lost it and now you must regain it. This is an individual path to take, one that is begun by many but followed through by few. It is your challenge to see if you can bring deeper dimensions to life consistently; to give your spirit fresh air to breathe while existing in a claustrophobic, material world that weighs it down. Sometimes the sharper this challenge, the greater the depth of learning. So don't give up because your world seems to be a crazy one built on fear and anxiety – this is to guide you in the opposite direction, reminding you where you do not want to be.

Your Challenge

The system of Reiki is for everyone, each child, teenager, adult and wise one can benefit from drawing more Ki through them to strengthen and cleanse their inner core. No matter what state the physical body is in – it can only be of benefit. The sense of connection that is experienced places its recipients in new light.

It is not so much about learning new things but about breaking down old patterns that have accumulated during your lifetime. By breaking away these habits you gradually discover your true nature.

Inherently, humanity has all the knowledge it needs.

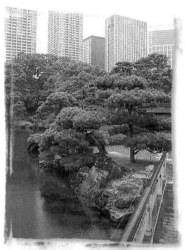

Once you have your routine you can then decide to add to it when you wish. Eventually this will come naturally to you without any pre-meditated thought at all. The concept of the living practice is that it is always with you. Think of ways to incorporate elements of the system into your everyday life – precept work, balance, strength, and healing abilities. This is the challenge set for you.

The *gokai* are there in your actions and with every word you speak. Just for today you are the five precepts.

Kokyû techniques strengthen your inner Ki so that you are no longer swayed so easily by what occurs around you. You learn to take back what is yours and develop it. This strengthened inner core allows you to purposefully extend your Ki or retract it in any situation.

Tenohira can be used at anytime, anyplace. If you are tired, place your hands on your *hara*. If your thumb is sore, cradle it in your other hand. When your head hurts, place one hand on your forehead and the other on the back of the skull. These natural movements receive extra benefit from your conscious application.

As you progress through the levels of the system of Reiki the *jumon* and *shirushi* teach you about Ki work, deepening your understanding of, and inner connection to, your path.

The receiving of *reiju* is there for everyone and its blessings shower down on both the performer and recipient. If you can receive *reiju* throughout life then this blessing will support your entire healing process.

Look at your anger and your worrying. Be humble, honest and compassionate. Breathe in and out with the flow of the universe and draw on your Ki for its higher purpose of healing. Finally, accept that all clearing is supported by the five elements and a healthy lifestyle. This is your chance to make whole again.

Appendices

Glossary of Japanese Words

Bokusen – divination
Chôbuku – exorcism
Dô – treatment, method or way
Enjudo – a hall for lengthening one's life, healing room found in a monastery
Enzui bu – either side of the neck
Gakkai – society
Gasshô – to place the two palms together
Gedoku – detoxification
Genki – spirit
Go shimbô – dharma for protecting the body, Tendai ritual
Gokai – five precepts
Gyô – ascetic practices
Gyosei – poetry (*waka*) written by the Emperor
Hara – belly or abdomen (also referred to as *tanden*)
Hatamoto – level of *samurai*, personal guard of the *shôgun*
Hatsurei – to generate greater amounts of spirit
Hiei zan – Mt Hiei near Kyôto, Japan

Hô – method
Hikkei – companion, manual
Hokkesen – the *Hokke* (relating to the Lotus Sutra) method of annulling sins
Honu no reikô – the spiritual light that exists within each person
Ichi-go, ich-e – one encounter, one opportunity
In – yin
Jôshin – focusing the mind
Jumon – spell or incantation, mantra
Kami – Shinto deity or god
Kanji – Japanese written characters
Kenyoku – dry bath
Kiriku – a seed syllable that calls upon the energy of Amida Nyorai
Kitô – incantation
Kokyû – breathing
Kosho michibiki – illuminating guidance, Eguchi's *reiju*
Kôtô bu – back of the head
Kotodama – words carrying spirit

Kurama yama – Mt Kurama near Kyôto, Japan

Manga – frivolous pictures, comics

Misogi – purification

Naga-iki – long breath

Nentatsu – sending thoughts

Nichirin in – sun mudra

Okuden – second stage

Reiju – offering of spiritual energy, blessing

Ryôhô – healing method

Samurai – warrior

Sansho – three times

Seishin – spirit, mind, soul, intention

Seiza – correct sitting

Sensei – teacher, master

Shihan – instructor or teacher

Shinpiden – mystery teachings

Shirushi – symbol

Shoden – first stage

Shôgun – general

Shugenja – those who accumulate spiritual power or experience, Shugendô practitioner

Sokutô bu – both temples

Tanden – below the navel (also referred to as *hara*)

Teate – hands-on healing (generic term)

Tenohira – palm-healing, using a specific structure

Tôchô bu – crown on head

Toitsu – to unite, unify (to make one)

Uchu-rei – universal mind

Wa – harmony

Waka – thirty-one syllable poem

Yamabushi – those who lie down in the mountains, Shugendô practitioner

Yo – yang

Zaike – lay priest

Zentô bu – front of the head

Japanese Reiki Precepts

The secret of inviting happiness through many blessings, the spiritual medicine for all illness

> For today only:
> Do not anger
> Do not worry
> Be humble
> Be honest in your work
> Be compassionate to yourself and others

Do *gasshô* every morning and evening, keep in your mind and recite
Improve your mind and body

Usui Reiki Ryôhô, the founder Usui Mikao

Translated by Chris Marsh.

Waka

Some *waka* have been included here for your interest and for you to incorporate into your practice. They can be used with either the *gokai* practices or *Hatsurei Hô*. These *waka* (originally written by the Meiji Emperor) have been taken from the *Reiki Ryôhô Hikkei*, a manual used by the *Usui Reiki Ryôhô Gakkai*. Inamoto Hyakuten translated these *waka*.

> *Akino yono tuskiwa mukashini kawaranedo*
> *yoni nakihito no ooku narinuru (Tsuki)*
> While a moon on an autumnal night remains just the same as ever,
> in this world the number of the deceased has become larger
> (Moon)

> *Asamidori sumiwataritaru ohzorano*
> *hiroki onoga kokoro to mogana (Ten)*
> As a great sky in clear light green
> I wish my heart would be as vast (Sky)

> *Atsushitomo iware zarikeri niekaeru*
> *mizutani tateru shizu wo omoheba (Orinifurete)*
> Thinking of lowly people standing in a boiling hot paddy field
> I hesitate to utter, 'It's hot' (upon occasion)

> *Amata tabi shigurete someshi momijiba wo*
> *tada hitokaze no chirashi kerukana (Rakuyou – fu)*
> Maple leaves tinted by frequent showers in late autumn
> just a whiff of wind scattered (Fallen Leaves – Wind)

Further Reading

Books are an invaluable source of information that can support and encourage your practice.

To further your personal understanding of the influences that formed the system of Reiki there are numerous books that might interest you. Some have been included below under their topic headings.

Shugendô:

Hitoshi Miyake. *Shugendô – Essays on the Structure of Japanese Folk Religion*, The University of Michigan, Michigan, 2001.

Shinto:

Breen, John and Mark Teeuwen. *Shinto in History – Ways of the Kami*, Curzon Press, Surrey, 2000.

Floyd, H. Ross. *Shinto: The Way of Japan*, Greenwood Publishing Group, Westport, 1965.

Martial Arts:

Funakoshi Gichin. *Karate-dô – My Way of Life*, Kodansha America Inc, New York, 1975.

Steven, John. *The Essence of Aikido*, Kodansha International, New York, 1999.

Tendai:

Groner, Paul. *Saicho – The Establishment of the Japanese Tendai School*, University of Hawaii Press, Honolulu, 2000.

Saso, Michael. *Tantric Art and Meditation*, Tendai Education

Foundation, Honolulu, 1990.

Watson, Burton. *The Lotus Sutra,* Columbia University Press, New York, 1993.

Japanese Buddhism:

Inagaki Hisao. *A Dictionary of Japanese Buddhist Terms,* Nagata Bunshodo, Kyôto, 2003.

Suzuki Shunryu. *Not Always So – Practicing the True Spirit of Zen,* HarperCollins, New York, 2002.

Meditation:

Suzuki Shunryu. *Zen Mind, Beginners Mind,* Weatherhill, New York, 1970.

Davey, H.E. *Living the Japanese Arts & Ways,* Stone Bridge Press, Berkeley, 2003.

Bibliography

Abé Ryûichi. *The Weaving of Mantra*, Columbia University Press, New York, 1999.

Ashton, W.G. (translated by) *The Nihongi*, 1896.

Bary De, WM Theodore. *Sources of Japanese Tradition*, Columbian University Press, New York, 2001.

Blacker, Carmen. *The Catalpa Bow – A Study of Shamanic Practices in Japan*, Japan Library, Richmond, 1999.

Breen, John and Mark Teeuwen. *Shinto in History – Ways of the Kami*, Curzon Press, Surrey, 2000.

Chadwick, David. *Thank You and Ok! An American Zen Failure in Japan*, Penguin Books, London, 1994.

Chadwick, David. *The Life and Zen Teachings of Shunryu Suzuki*, Thorsons, London, 1999.

Cleary, Thomas. *The Japanese Art of War – Understanding the Culture of Strategy*, Shambhala Publications, Boston, 1991.

Cleary, Thomas. *The Book of Five Rings*, Shambhala Publications, Boston, 1994.

Cleary, Thomas. *The Code of the Samurai – A Contemporary Translation of the Bushido Shoshinshu of Taira Shigesuke*, Tuttle Publishing, Boston, 2000.

Cleary, Thomas. *The Inner Teachings of Taoism*, Shambhala Publications, Boston, 1986.

Davey, H.E. *Living the Japanese Arts & Ways*, Stone Bridge Press, Berkeley, 2003.

Davey, H.E. *Japanese Yoga – The Way of Dynamic Meditation*, Stone Bridge Press, Berkeley, 2001.

Doi Hiroshi. *Modern Reiki Method for Healing*, Fraser Journal Publishing, British Columbia, 2000.

Eguchi Toshihiro. *Te No Hira Ryôji Nyûmon*, Arusu Publishing, Japan, 1930.

Eguchi Toshihiro. *Te No Hira Ryôji Dokuhon*, Kaikosha Publishing, Japan 1936.

Eguchi Toshihiro. *Te No Hira Ryôji Wo Kataru*, Japan, 1954.

Floyd, H. Ross. *Shinto: The Way of Japan*, Greenwood Publishing Group, Westport, 1965.

Funakoshi Gichin. *Karate-dô – My Way of Life*, Kodansha America Inc, New York, 1975.

Gordon, Andrew. *A Modern History of Japan: From Tokugawa Times to the Present*, Oxford University Press, Oxford, 2002.

Groner, Paul. *Saicho – The Establishment of the Japanese Tendai School*, University of Hawaii Press, Honolulu, 2000.

Hadamitzky, Wolfgang and Spahn, Mark. *Kanji & Kana – A Handbook and Dictionary of the Japanese Writing System*, Tuttle Publishing, Boston, 1981.

Hanh, Thich Nhat. *Opening the Heart of the Cosmos – Insights on the Lotus Sutra*, Paralax Press, Berkeley, 2003.

Hanh, Thich Nhat. *The Diamond that Cuts Through Illusion – Commentaries on the Prajnaparamita Diamond Sutra*, SCB Distributors, Gardena, 1992.

Hayashi Chûjirô. *Ryôhô Shishin*, Japan.

Herrigel, Eugen. *Zen in the Art of Archery*, Vintage, London, 1999.

Hitoshi Miyake. *Shugendô – Essays on the Structure of Japanese Folk Religion*, The University of Michigan, Michigan, 2001.

Honna Nobuyuki and Hoffer, Bates. *An English Dictionary of Japanese Culture*, Yuhikaku Publishing Co. Ltd. Tôkyô, 1986.

Ikeda Mitsuru (translated by Andrew Driver). *The World of the Hotsuma Legends*, Japan Translation Center, Tôkyô, 1996.

Ikegami Eiko. *The Taming of the Samurai: Honorific Individualism and the Making of Modern Japan*, Harvard University Press, Cambridge, 1995.

Irie Taikichi and Aoyama, Shigery (translated by Thomas I. Elliott). *Buddhist Images*, Hoikusha Publishing Co Ltd. Osaka, 1999.

Inagaki Hisao. *A Dictionary of Japanese Buddhist Terms*, Nagata Bunshodo, Kyôto, 2003.

Japanese Journals of Religious Studies, Nanzan Institute for Religion and Culture, Japan.

Kamalashila. *Meditation – The Buddhist Way of Tranquility and Insight*, Windhorse Publications, Glasgow, 1992.

Keene, Donald. *Emperor of Japan – Meiji and His World, 1852–1912*, Columbia University Press, New York, 2002.

Kohno Jiko. *Right View, Right Life*, Kosei Publishing Co, Tôkyô, 1998.

LaFleur, William R. *The Karma of Words – Buddhism and the Literary Arts in Medieval Japan*, University of California Press, Los Angeles, 1986.

Nishida Tenko. *A New Road To Ancient Truth*, Horizon Press, New York, 1972.

Maruyana Koretsohi. *Aikidô with Ki, Ki-no-Kenkyûkai*, Tôkyô, 1984.

Matsumoto Yoshinosuke (translated by Andrew Driver). *An Unknown History of Ancient Japan, The Hotsuma Legends – Paths of the Ancestors*, Japan Translation Center, Tôkyô, 1999.

McCarthy, Patrick and Yukio. *Funakoshi Gichin's Tanpenshu*, International Ryukyu Karate Research Society, Brisbane, 2002.

Mihashi Kazuo. *Tenohira-ga Byoki-o Naosu*, Chuo Art Publishing Co, Ltd. Japan, 2001.

Mizutani, Osamu and Nobuku. *An Introduction to Modern Japanese*, Japan Times Ltd, Tôkyô, 1977.

Mochizuki Toshitaka. *Iyashi No Te, Tama Shuppan*, Tôkyô, 1995.

Mochizuki Toshitaka. *Chô Kantan Iyashi No Te*, Tama Shuppan, Tôkyô, 2001.

Murumoto, Wayne. 'What is a Ryu?' Issue 8, *Furyu-The Budo Journal*, Tengu Press, Hawaii.

Nelson, Andrew N. *The Modern Reader's Japanese-English Character Dictionary*, Tuttle Publishing, Boston, 1972.

Oda Ryuko. *Kaji – Empowerment and Healing in Esoteric Buddhism*, Kineizan Shinjao-in Mitsumonkai, Japan, 1992.

Papinot, Edmond. *Historical and Geographical Dictionary of Japan*, Tuttle Publishing, Boston, 1972.

Petter, Frank Arjava. *Reiki Fire*, Lotus Press, Twin Lakes, 1998.

Reed, William. *Ki – A Practical Guide for Westerners*, Japan Publications Inc, Tôkyô, 1986.

Reiki Ryôhô Hikkei, Usui Reiki Ryôhô Gakkai, Japan.

Sargent, Jiho. *Asking About Zen – 108 Answers*, Weatherhill, Inc. New

York, 2001.

Saso, Michael. *Tantric Art and Meditation*, Tendai Education Foundation, Honolulu, 1990.

Steven, John. *Sacred Calligraphy of the East*, Shambhala Publications, Boston, 1996.

Steven, John. *The Essence of Aikido*, Kodansha International, New York, 1999.

Steven, John. *The Marathon Monks of Mount Hiei*, Shambhala Publications, Boston 1988.

Stiene, Bronwen and Frans. *The Reiki Sourcebook*, O Books, Winchester, 2003.

Suzuki D.T. *Buddha of Infinite Light – The Teachings of Shin Buddhism, The Japanese Way of Wisdom and Compasion*, Shambhala Publications, Boston, 1998.

Suzuki Shunryu. *Zen Mind, Beginners Mind*, Weatherhill, New York, 1970.

Suzuki Shunryu. *Branching Streams Flow in the Darkness: Lectures on the Sandokai*, University of California Press, Berkeley, 1999.

Suzuki Shunryu. *Not Always So – Practicing the True Spirit of Zen*, HarperCollins, New York, 2002.

Tanabe, George J. Jr. *Religions of Japan in Practice*, Princeton University Press, Princeton, 1999.

The Encyclopedia of Eastern Philosophy and Religion, Shambhala Publications, Boston, 1994.

Tohei Koichi. *Ki in Daily Life*, Ki-no-Kenkyûkai, Tôkyô, 1980.

Tohei Koichi. *Book of Ki- Coordinating Mind and Body in Daily Life*, Japan Publications Inc, Tôkyô, 1976.

Tomita Kaiji. *Reiki To Jinjutsu – Tomita Ryû Teate Ryôhô*, BAB Japan, Tôkyô, 1999.

Unno Taitetsu. *River of Fire – River of Water – An Introduction to the Pure Land Tradition of Shin Buddhism*, Doubleday, New York, 1998.

Varley, Paul. *Japanese Culture* (Fourth Edition), University of Hawai'i Press, Honolulu, 2000.

Watson, Burton. *The Lotus Sutra*, Columbia University Press, New York, 1993.

Yun, Hsing. *Lotus in a Stream*, Weatherhill, Inc. Trumbull, 2000.

Notes

Part I

[1] *The Formation of Sect Shinto* by Inoue Mobutaka. Japanese Journal of Religious Studies 29/3-4, Nanzan Institute for Religion and Culture, Nagoya, 2002.

[2] *Shugendô* by Miyake Hitoshi. Center for Japanese Studies, The University of Michigan, Ann Arbor, MI, 2001.

[3] For more information about the attunement and *reiju* see Chapter 9, Part II.

[4] Information supplied to the authors by Suzuki san's aide and translator.

[5] The term esoteric is used in Buddhism, martial arts and the New Age movement. Depending on the context it is used in it will refer to different practices. Even within Buddhism the term will be used to represent something different depending on the branch.

[6] The Lotus Sutra is one of the most important texts of Mahayana Buddhism and is believed to include the complete teachings of Gautama Buddha.

[7] *Japanese Culture* (4th edition) by Paul Varley, University of Hawai'i Press, Honolulu, 2000.

[8] *Zen in the Art of Archery* by Eugen Herrigel, Random House, 1999.

[9] *Japanese Culture* (4th edition) by Paul Varley, University of Hawai'i Press, Honolulu, 2000.

[10] Information supplied to the authors by Suzuki san's aide and translator.

[11] *Sensei* is an honorific name for teacher. One may not call one's self a *sensei* as it is a sign of respect shown by others.

[12] Information supplied to the authors by Chris Marsh.

[13] Information supplied to the authors by Professor Judith Rabinovitch.

Ph.D., Harvard University; Currently Karashima Professor of Japanese Language and Culture Department of Foreign Languages and Literature, University of Montana, USA. She studied *tenohira ryôji* with Miss Endo (an original *Ittôen* student of Eguchi) for one week in 1974 at the *Ittôen* community in Japan and received an informal initiation where Miss Endo, sitting quietly in a state of meditation, placed her hands upon hers while in contact with the student for about one hour, advising her to keep practising. Rabinovitch reports feeling great energy in her body and hands thereafter and continued to practice for 10 years. She went on to train through to the teacher level with a Japanese priest in 2002.

[14] Information supplied to the authors by Chris Marsh.

[15] *Living the Japanese Arts and Ways* by H.E. Davey, Stone Bridge Press, Berkeley, 2003.

[16] Information supplied to the authors by Chris Marsh.

[17] Shamans in Japan, according to Carmen Blacker author of *The Catalpa Bow*, believe in paradise. They have the ability to communicate with this 'other world'. Their gifts include the power of healing and clairvoyance that 'contact with the sacred often bestows'.

[18] *Shugendô* by Miyake Hitoshi, Center for Japanese Studies, The University of Michigan, 2001.

[19] *Shugendô* by Miyake Hitoshi, Center for Japanese Studies, The University of Michigan, 2001.

[20] Some of Usui's students (an association called the *Usui Reiki Ryôhô Gakkai*) engraved and mounted the memorial stone in 1927, one year after Usui's death. For a complete translation by Inamoto Hyakuten see *The Reiki Sourcebook* by Bronwen and Frans Stiene.

[21] The Saihôji Temple is located at Toyotama District, 1–4–56 Umesato, Suginami Ku, Tôkyô.

[22] *The Catalpa Bow* by Carmen Blacker, Japan Library, Richmond, 1999.

[23] *Shugendô* by Miyake Hitoshi, Center for Japanese Studies, The University of Michigan.

[24] From a teaching given by Chris Marsh in Belgium, 2003.

[25] A Sect is a group adhering to a distinctive doctrine.

[26] Information supplied to the authors by Suzuki san's aide and translator.

[27] *Japanese Culture* (4th edition) by Paul Varley, University of Hawai'i Press, Honolulu, 2000.

[28] For an English translation of a list of Japanese *tenohira* groups see *The Reiki Sourcebook* under 'Reiki in Japan' by Bronwen and Frans Stiene.

[29] *The Catalpa Bow* by Carmen Blacker, Japan Library, Richmond, 1999.

[30] *Reiki Fire* by Frank Arjava Petter, Lotus Press, Twin Lakes, 1998.

[31] Information supplied to the authors by Professor Judith Rabinovitch. Ph.D., Harvard University; Currently Karashima Professor of Japanese Language and Culture Department of Foreign Languages and Literature, University of Montana, USA.

[32] The authors interviewed Yamaguchi Chiyoko and her son Tadao in Kyôto in 2001.

[33] Hayashi Chie was spoken of by both Yamaguchi Chiyoko and Hawayo Takata.

[34] Dave King claims to have met a person called Tatsumi who was a teacher student of Hayashi Chûjirô.

[35] Information supplied to the authors by Yamaguchi Chiyoko, 2001.

[36] A Lineage is a list of teachers tracing back to the founder of the system. A lineage can indicate what information and methods are being passed on to a student.

[37] *Shugendô* by Miyake Hitoshi, Center for Japanese Studies, The University of Michigan.

Part II

[1] Translation by Chris Marsh.

[2] For a full copy of the Japanese precepts see the Appendices.

[3] Information supplied to the authors by Chris Marsh.

[4] For more translations of the Meiji Emperor's *waka* see the Appendices.

[5] Many techniques have been added since the system came to the West. In Japan, even a traditional society such as the *Usui Reiki Ryôhô Gakkai* has a wide variety of techniques listed in their manual or *Hikkei* that have been added to over the years.

[6] *Ki – A Practical Guide for Westerners* by William Reed, Japan Publications Inc, Tokyo, 1986.

[7] *Waka* translation is copyright Inamoto Hyakuten.

[8] Information supplied to the authors by Chris Marsh.

[9] *Living the Japanese Arts and Ways* by H.E. Davey, Stone Bridge Press, Berkeley, California, 2003.

[10] Information supplied to the authors by Chris Marsh.

[11] Information from Doi Hiroshi.

[12] Information supplied to the authors by Chris Marsh.

[13] Information supplied to the authors by Chris Marsh.

[14] Stylized letterforms used for meditation in Eastern cultures.

[15] *The Essence of Aikido* compiled by John Stevens, Kodansha International, Tôkyô, 1993.

[16] *Kanji* are Japanese written characters.

[17] Translation by Doi Hiroshi.

[18] *The Inner Teachings of Taoism* by Chang Po-Tuan translated by Thomas Cleary, Shambhala Publications, Boston, 1986.

[19] Information supplied to the authors by Chris Marsh.

[20] *The Lotus Sutra* by Burton Watson, Columbia University Press, New York, 1993.

Index

192   *The Japanese Art of Reiki*